Optimizing Schizophrenia!

(Because Schizophrenics' Lives Matter)

By

Chris O Hapinez

Published in 2022

Contents

TOPIC	page
Preface	7
A Healthy Lifestyle	9
Anti-psychotics – relative adverse effects	15
Benefits Advice	17
Benefits/Work	18
Books	20
Chess	38
Cognitive Behavioural Therapy	39
Cognitive Remediation Therapy	40
Concessionary Schemes that may apply	41
Confidence Building	42
Depression	43
Dietary help for schizophrenics and perhaps others	45
Dose-Response Curve for Me (Estimated)	46
Famous Schizophrenics	48
Films	49
Food supplements for schizophrenics	53
General Mental Health	54

Group Homes	55
Half-Life of Anti-psychotic Medication	56
Heartland	58
Influence on weight of various drugs	59
Information from the World Wide Web	60
James Middleton	61
Links between Schizophrenia, Autism and Bipolar Disorder	62
Medication Side Effects	63
Mind Leaflets	64
Mystery Shoppers	65
Notorious Treatment of Schizophrenics in Nazi Germany	66
Notorious treatment of the mentally ill in the past and present even in the UK and US!	67
Notorious treatment of troublesome citizens as if mentally ill	68
Opportunities to be a service-user researcher/service user expert	69
Optimizing Schizophrenia	70

Organizations	74
Other uses of drugs used for schizophrenia	78
Personal Note	81
Photography	82
Plays	83
Prejudice in the Workplace	84
Problems which are more likely to arise in children of schizophrenics	85
Psychoeducation	86
Psychosis	87
Publications for schizophrenics and others	88
Publishers Dealing With Mental Health Topics	89
Radio Programmes on Madness	90
Reducing Medication	91
Reducing Medication II	96
Reducing Medication III	108
Religion	124
Research	125
Schizophrenia Caused by Illegal Drugs	139
Schizophrenia Journals	140

Service Users' Experiences	141
Smoking	142
Stress	143
Symbols to look out for when seeking an employer	145
Symptoms	146
The Author's Relevant Mathematical Ideas	147
The Law	158
The Madness and Genius/Creativity Connection	159
Therapeutic Art	160
Treatment for Schizophrenia	161
Treatment without Drugs	162
Understanding Schizophrenia	163
Universal Credit	164
University Life	165
Websites on schizophrenia and other mental illnesses and quotes from the web	166
Weight gain with antipsychotics	170
Work Capability Assessments	171
What can aid or prevent recovery	172

What some psychology students

were taught about schizophrenia					179

Preface

This book is an attempt to help ensure people with schizophrenia live a life that is as good as possible, i.e., they have an *optimal* experience of schizophrenia. There are many factors that help towards achieving this goal. Having good insight into one's illness is generally very important and the section *The Author's Relevant Mathematical Ideas* is potentially life-changing for some in this respect. Arguably of next most importance is making sure the dose given of some antipsychotic is chosen to enable *optimal* and not just adequate functioning. Hence the sections *Optimizing Schizophrenia, Dose-Response Curve for Me (Estimated), Reducing Medication, Reducing Medication II* and *Reducing Medication III* are key.

This book summarises what the author has learnt about schizophrenia and other mental illnesses. Sources are mentioned whenever possible but the treatment of the subject of schizophrenia is not meant to be at all comprehensive. Indeed, many topics (all listed in alphabetical order) are touched upon very briefly. There are many other books which give basic facts about schizophrenia which can be referred to in order to round out one's knowledge of it, some of which are mentioned in this book. Here I am simply trying to convey to others with schizophrenia (and/or their friends and relatives) the bits of relevant knowledge I have gleaned from various sources during the years 2000 to 2022 and accelerate their psychoeducation, in the hope that the sufferer may recover more quickly and fully. I have not attempted to make the book comprehensive as I think I have probably spent enough time learning about mental illnesses and it is time for me to direct most of my attention to other matters.

Some words of warning: many of the facts about schizophrenia in this book make grim reading. I hope it does not depress you too much if you or someone you know has schizophrenia. However, I thought it better that you be informed rather than remain ignorant. In addition, sufferers of schizophrenia should consult their psychiatrist before altering any dose of medication.

A Healthy Lifestyle

Eating healthily, exercising regularly, sleeping well etc. can help your mood and mental state generally.

Regarding exercise, you may be able to get a discount on sport and leisure activities if you are receiving benefits.

Given that schizophrenics die at least 25 years sooner than normal people on average, it might be an idea to consider the following summary.

From Daily Express, Monday December 29th 2008:

Ways to add on years or lose years of life:

Add on years:

+8 years for being an optimist.

+7 years for having faith.

+7 years for having an active mind.

+4 years for having good sex.

+2 years if you have a good view from your window.

+2 years if you keep your home safe.

+2 years if you own a pet.

+1 year if you nap in the afternoon.

Lose years:

-7 years for being a couch potato.

-5 years for thinking "I'm too old".

-4 years for having a bad doctor.

-4 years for fast food addiction.

-3 years for being obese.

-2 years for having a bad posture.

-2 years for being stressed.

-1 year for living with clutter.

-1 year for being underweight.

From The Guardian, *Old age starts at 80 as brains keep getting younger*, by Tim Radford:

Ancient Romans had a life expectancy of 22.

A seven-point plan to ensure a youthful old age is:

Keep aerobic fitness levels good.

Mental stimulation is vital.

New learning is important.

Avoid high and prolonged stress.

Seek a rich social life.

Eat healthily.

Think young.

<u>Helping the Brain</u>

Given the cognitive impairment in 85% of schizophrenics, the following might be of interest:

From New Scientist, 28th May 2005, '11 steps to a better brain':

1. Smart Drugs – drugs like Modafinil and Ritalin may help the brain stay awake and concentration respectively, but little is known about the effects of long term use and they may not be suitable for schizophrenics. However, dozens of others are being developed and maybe some will work to help schizophrenics overcome cognitive impairment.

    N.B. In Schizophrenia Bulletin, Volume 31, Number 2, April 2005, p.501 is an abstract entitled 'A double-blind placebo controlled trial of modafinil for negative symptoms in schizophrenia'

    From New Scientist, 14th May 2005, p. 6-7:

    Brain-boosters called ampakines work by boosting the activity of glutamate, a key neurotransmitter that makes it easier to learn and encode memory. Cortex produces an ampakine called CX717 which it is considering as a possible treatment for, among other illnesses, Alzheimer's disease.

2. Food for thought – have a breakfast, high fibre and protein is good. Omelette and salad plus yoghurt for pudding is good for lunch. Fish for the evening meal including strawberries and blueberries for pudding.
3. Various technical short-cuts may help the brain such as transcranial magnetic stimulation (TMS) though perhaps they're not readily available to many.
4. Train your working memory.
5. Learn a few tips from the contenders at the world memory championships – place items to be remembered along a visualised route.

6. Get a good night's sleep.
7. Get plenty of exercise – muscular work exercises the grey matter too.
8. Nuns on a run – the nuns on Good Counsel Hill in Mankato, Minnesota live especially long lives. Activities such as crosswords, knitting and exercising helped to prevent senility. The old adage "use it or lose it" is pertinent.
9. Focus attention – anything that raises dopamine levels can boost your powers of concentration. One way of doing this is caffeine but if you prefer the drug-free approach, the best strategy is to sleep well, eat foods packed with slow-release sugars, and take lots of exercise.
10. Engage in neurofeedback.

From The Guardian, 22.7.14, page 33, Students focus on high performance: "... Sahakian replied that research on patients with schizophrenia had shown that Modafinil not only helped "cold cognition" – such as memory, problem-solving and planning – but also "hot cognition" – emotional and social functions, such as recognising the expressions on people's faces."

According to Luton and Dunstable's *Herald & Post*, date unknown, oily fish, plenty of water, a small amount of caffeine (say one or two cups of tea or coffee daily), dark chocolate and soya foods are all good for the brain.

The adage "use it or lose it" seems to have much truth in it. Keeping our minds active seems to protect against Alzheimer's disease because it develops 'cognitive reserve', according to New Scientist, 17th December 2005, p. 32-35.

For good health it is best to avoid smoking, alcohol, non-prescription drugs, fat or sugar. It is good to have plenty of fibre, fruit, vegetables, complex carbohydrates, some protein and oily fish and plenty of water. It is also important to exercise regularly for at least 30 minutes at least 3 times a week, sleep well, and exercise your brain too.

For more on the link between smoking cannabis and developing schizophrenia, see New Scientist, 26th March 2005, p. 44-47.

I reckon if you live to 100 years old you have probably had a fairly healthy lifestyle, so if you want to look after yourself and get advice on how to do this better, check out the life expectancy calculator on the website http://www.livingto100.com .

Often, according to Rethink, the physical healthcare of the mentally ill is neglected, so look after yourself!

The New Economics Foundation says the five foundation stones of wellbeing are: connect, be active, take notice, keep learning and give.

The Health Education Authority in 1999 gave the following Positive Steps for Mental Health: Accepting who you are, Talking about it, Keeping active, Learning new skills, Keeping in touch with friends, Doing something creative, Getting involved, Asking for help, Relaxing, Surviving.

The booklet "How to … Look after your mental health" by The Mental Health Foundation lists 10 things to do:

1. Talk about your feelings
2. Keep active
3. Eat well
4. Drink sensibly
5. Keep in touch
6. Ask for help
7. Take a break
8. Do something you're good at
9. Accept who you are
10. Care for others

Anti-psychotics – relative adverse effects

From the National Schizophrenia Fellowship (now called Rethink):

Drug	Sedation	Extra-Pyramidal	Potential for Cardio-toxicity	Prolactin elevation	Weight gain
Chlorpromazine	+++	++	++	+++	++
Promazine	+++	+	+	++	++
Thioridazine	+++	+	+++	++	+++
Fluphenazine	+	+++	+	+++	+
Perphenazine	+	+++	+	+++	+
Trifluoperazine	+	+++	+	+++	+
Flupenthixol	+	++	+	+++	++
Zuclopenthixol	++	++	+	+++	++
Haloperidol	+	+++	+	+++	+
Benperidol	+	+++	+	+++	+
Sulpiride	-	+	-	+++	+
Pimozide	+	+	+++	+++	+

Loxapine	++	+++	+	+++	+
Clozapine	+++	-	+	-	+++
Risperidone	+	+	-	+++	++
Olanzapine	++	+/-	-	+	+++
Quetiapine	++	-	-	-	++
Amisulpride	-	+	-	+++	+
Zotepine	+++	++	++	++	+++

Key   +++ High incidence/severity

++ Moderate   + Low   - Very low

Benefits Advice

One possible source of advice and help regarding benefits is your local Citizens Advice Bureau.

Benefits/Work

From The Observer, 19.09.10: article titled: *"Jobless are as happy as those in work"*: It is not what a government determined to get people off benefits wants to hear, but a study has thrown cold water on the idea that those who don't work are less happy than those that do.

New research has found that although the jobless are generally less satisfied with their lot than people in work, their day-to-day emotional wellbeing remains the same. The paradox, identified by a group of German economists, is published in this week's Economic Journal.

Their study is the first to use the "day reconstruction method" developed by Nobel economics laureate, Daniel Kahneman, that combines a time-use survey with the empirical measurement of people's happiness. A total of 600 employed and unemployed respondents were asked to construct a diary of the previous day, listing all the activities they engaged in and how they felt during each one.

In line with previous research, the study found unemployed people are less satisfied with their life in general. But when it comes to their emotions on a specific day, the unemployed have the same average level of positive and negative feelings as the employed. Or, as the title of the study explains, the unemployed are "dissatisfied with life, but having a good day".

The authors note: "Whether people are in a job or not, they almost all report being happiest during leisure time. The employed, however, are least happy when at work or commuting. Since the unemployed can spend that time on leisure, their unemployment hurts much less emotionally than previously thought."

From The Daily Express, 24.10.17, p. 13, by Vanessa Feltz:

"Ministers believe all 10-year olds should be given career advice. They're right and here it is. Very few people are lucky enough to make their hobby their job. Most jobs are repetitive, boring in parts and involve spending time in a place you'd rather not be, sitting in close proximity to people you'd rather not know. Nevertheless, as long as it doesn't damage your health, a job is a great thing. With it you have a framework, social interaction, a level of respect and a pay cheque. Without it you have freedom but no funds and an infinite capacity to waste time and end up in trouble.

Stop gilding the lily. We can't all be captains of industry or David Beckham. Tell 10-year-olds the stark but bracing truth."

Books

Books I have read:

Abnormal Psychology by Philip Kendall and Constance Hammen:

I found this book very helpful in understanding a range of mental illnesses.

Me, Myself, and Them by Kurt Snyder with Raquel Gur and Linda Wasmer Andrews:

I read an earlier version of this with a different title, I think.

The Soloist by Steve Lopez:

I was given the book "The Soloist" after seeing the film of the same name (see film section). The story is similar to, but naturally more informative than, the film, and, surprisingly, also more upbeat than the film as it seems Nathaniel has functioned a little better than he was depicted as doing in the film. However, I won't spoil it for you by saying in what way. I can recommend both the book and the film.

Staying Sane by Dr Raj Persaud:

p. 47, para 2: "Another key aspect of having many purposes, or a deep purpose, in life is that this means there are things for which you are prepared to endure personal sacrifice. Learning to tolerate and endure negative experience for ends you consider worthwhile is also a vital part of positive mental health."

p. 47, end of para 3: "So we may begin to learn to control our temper, not when our family complains about it, but only when we realise our tantrums are putting our pay-rise at work in jeopardy."

p. 134, end of para 5: "The surest way to end up needing to see a mental health professional is to have things in your life you need to share, confess or discuss, but not to have anyone with whom you can do it."

p. 148, beginning of para 2: "In each of these examples, as in much of poor mental health, too much self-worth has become centred on one particular aspect of life."

p. 162, beginning of para 5: "An interesting paradox of the comfort zone thus emerges, in that an individual's psychological strength lies not in avoiding negative judgements by others, but in a willingness to confront the risk of appraisal."

p. 167, end of para 7: "Any success that does not require personal growth is probably a success born of setting our sights too low."

p. 168, para 3: "You need to insulate yourself against poor mental health by ensuring greater self-complexity so that poor performances, untoward events or losses in one sphere of life, do not produce catastrophic collapses in feelings of self-worth."

p. 178, beginning of para 6: "One of the best ways of preventing depression is to ensure that important rewards come from more than one source."

p. 199, part of para 6: "So, again paradoxically, more intelligent people are likely to feel bored."

p. 200, part of para 2: "The ability to focus and concentrate mitigates against boredom."

p. 203, end of para 4: "If your own attempts to cheer yourself up are failing, so that nothing at all seems to give you pleasure or lifts your mood, it is likely you need to see a specialist."

p. 206, part of para 2: "Anxiety and depression so often co-exist that it is difficult to distinguish them from each other."

p. 209, end of para 4: "being able to distract yourself from the cause of your bad mood (or the mood itself) is a crucial mental health skill. Psychologists often call this 'emotional management'."

p. 239, beginning of para 5: "Research has also shown that feeling good helps our problem-solving ability."

p. 240, para 3: "Although distraction and problem-solving appear to be opposite approaches, positive mental health means having both available to you, and knowing when to switch your strategy as the situation demands."

p. 252, beginning of para 5: "The most mature defences of all are humour and sublimation which imply an ability to accept difficult situations, while taking the edge off pain by producing a creative response to anxiety."

p. 258, beginning of para 5: "Some symptoms of mental disorders are physical, and include loss of weight, palpitations, tingling in the limbs and nausea."

p. 270, end of para 2: "For example, while having a high IQ as a child seems to be of general benefit while the going is non-stressful, there is some evidence that, in the face of adversity, children with high IQs do worse in some circumstances than those with lower IQs."

p. 275, para 6: "The reason why long-term goals are crucial to mental health is that ambitions drive you forward and so often put you in situations where you have to do things you would rather not do. You do them in order to attain your long-term aspirations."

p. 284, beginning of para 2: "If you wish to be mentally healthy, you must judge your reactions carefully to make sure you are not over-reacting."

p. 292, end of para 6: "It seems that the more upbeat you are, the more it helps protect your mental health."

p. 315, end of para 2: "Coping is like a muscle, the more you use it, the stronger it becomes, whereas if you determine not to use it, it atrophies."

p. 337, part of para 2: "... this reduction in hippocampal volume has been found in depressed people who had been exposed to less extreme situations and had never been in war."

A Beautiful Mind by Sylvia Nasar:

This is a biography of John Forbes Nash Jr., on which the film with the same name is based.

Eyebrows & Other Fish by Anthony Scally:

This book, available from the site www.lulu.com is about the author's experience of Schizophrenia. The author says he does not hear voices but certainly suffers from paranoia and delusions of reference at times. The author integrates autobiographical information with the schizophrenia-related story and has had relationship difficulties, suffers childhood abuse and he only has a proper job for a short time before succumbing to the illness. Despite this he does later get married and has children. However, this is not a tale of triumph over adversity and wonderful recovery and achievement despite illness (as the film A Beautiful Mind was

23

supposed to be). Instead it is a story of a comparatively normal and ordinary person who develops schizophrenia and, like most of the sufferers of this illness, does not fully recover. He does, however, play a leading role for a time in trying to make people aware of the illness in a less negative way than is often portrayed in the media. It appears to be quite open and honest about the author and does not hide the unpleasant things that happen in his life. I found that this story brought home to me the fragility of the mental health of some people with schizophrenia and made me feel fortunate that my experiences of schizophrenia in hospital and outside have not been too bad. Everyone's experience of schizophrenia is different, just as everyone's life is different and if, like me, you are interested in reading another (fairly young, British) person's story, written by the sufferer, then I expect you will be pleased to read this book. It is available as a download (£2.84 at time of purchase) as well as in print form (£9.99 paperback).

Living with Schizophrenia by John Watkins:

p. 7, para 2, line 4: "In fact, these drugs may sometimes contribute to a worsening of problems such as slowness and lack of motivation" (c.f. dopamine is a motivator)

p.22, para 4, line 5: "the side effects of neuroleptic medications sometimes contribute to negative symptoms such as loss of motivation or emotional flatness".

Schizophrenia the facts by Ming T. Tsuang and Stephen V. Faraone:

"Schizophrenics have deficits in immediate attention, sustained attention and selective attention, also abstraction and concept formation, and left side of brain (governing thought & language), also verbal ability, language, learning and memory. They fare better, however, on spatial tasks, such as memorizing & reproducing specified patterns, objects shapes or forms."

Authentic Happiness by Martin E.P. Seligman

The Centre Cannot Hold by Elyn R. Saks:

This is an autobiography of someone who works in a high-powered job despite having schizophrenia. It was mentioned on Radio 4.

This book is the autobiography of a Professor in the United States who has succeeded in getting degrees, holding down her busy role as a professor and getting married despite suffering from schizophrenia. Unlike so many who do their best work before getting the illness, she has triumphed and received some honours from her university after getting her illness. She has had many psychological crises, and feels that psychoanalysis has helped her greatly. Some of the tales of her psychoanalysis, especially with a Kleinian analyst in Oxford, are fascinating and it is interesting to contrast the approach by hospital staff in the U.S., where physical restraints are used liberally, with that in the U.K. where they are not used. I think Elyn Saks can now be considered one of my heroines, achieving significant things intellectually despite so many troubles, mostly mental, but also including a couple of cancers. In summary, I found this book to be a real page-turner and the best read I have had in about ten years.

Schizophrenia: A very short introduction by Christopher Frith & Eve Johnstone.

Our Voices: First-Person Accounts of Schizophrenia Edited by Colette Corr et al.

Delusions of Grandeur by Talmadge Rogalla:

Like it says on the back cover, this book is written in a creative and fluid style, so it is a pleasant and easy read. It is fiction, with lots of dialogue and description and mirrors the author's own experiences of psychosis. The book starts with the main character, Friedrich, in a psychiatrist's room telling the tale of what happened to him. He says he was contacted by an angel and began to believe that he is a special person whose destiny is to save mankind from nuclear destruction. We are led to believe that he has adventures with the army and they help him realise his goal with the help of technology and the special cup given to him by the angel. However, if I interpreted it right, it seems in the end all this was just hallucinations and delusions and Friedrich is really psychotic and has to take pills for his illness. There is an amusing ending. I think the author could have done better in 'educating the reader about psychotic thought' as it claims on the back cover, but I also think it is quite well written and a reasonable purchase if you want something that might be called 'schizo-fiction'.

Frank: Fighting Back by Frank Bruno with Kevin Mitchell.

Defender: Adventures in Schizophrenia by Richard M Clements:

If you want to know the thoughts of someone who is very mad, this could be the book for you. The book is essentially an autobiography but the author has lived in a world of his own psychotic imagination to such an extent and for so long that it seems more like fiction. It reminds me of a science fiction book I abandoned reading in my youth because it introduced too many made-up words, but perhaps this is a book of great value to psychologists. The author suffers voices with his schizophrenia and seems to me to have been very ill. The book is clever, creative and full of complex fantasies and delusions, extraordinary and amazing concepts and ideas imagined due to psychosis. On the other hand, one could describe the book as mostly psychotic ramblings and extremely difficult to fathom. Indeed, I found it grows tiresome after a while reading almost nonsense and understanding just fragments of it. Whilst reading it I was longing for him to get well and start making sense. Eventually, he does get a bit better, but still hears voices and lives in sheltered accommodation. If you are interested, it could be worth getting this book for the extraordinary 'mind-life' it contains.

Autobiography of a Schizophrenic Girl: The True Story of "Renee":

This is a book by someone who received psychotherapy for their schizophrenia.

One Flew Over the Cuckoo's Nest by Ken Kesey:

This is an excellent fictional story. I bought this book for £2.99 a few years ago from HMV (of all places) and didn't read it till I saw it was listed under the best novels about madness section of "1000 Novels Everyone Must Read" in The Guardian. It is a fine novel in my opinion too, and nearly all of it is believable (to me at least) as something that could have happened in early sixties America when it was published in 1962. I had already seen the film version, and the book added considerably to my knowledge from the film. It tells the story of life in a mental institution in America in the middle of the 20th Century. The narrator, Chief Bromden, who has been in the hospital or a previous one for many years naturally features a lot more in the novel and he can mix with some of the staff on occasion because he pretends to be, and is thought to be, deaf and dumb. This enables the staff's behaviour to be described too. New patient Randle Patrick McMurphy (played by Jack Nicholson in the film) immediately has a huge impact on the ward, dominating affairs there with his gambling and fighting ways, changing and building up the confidence of the patients - especially Chief Bromden. This aspect is missed out in the film, as far as I remember, along with, for example, a fight in which McMurphy and Chief Bromden beat up a couple of the black aides and end up in a "Disturbed Ward", which despite its name was potentially a better place for him than the original ward because it is not run by the dreaded, all-powerful and controlling, Nurse Ratched. There is a long-running battle between McMurphy and Ratched, which has a similar, but interestingly different, ending from the film. Well worth a read, I think.

Exuberance: The Passion for Life by Kay Redfield Jamison:

This is a bipolar-disorder-related book by a famous author and sufferer of bipolar disorder.

An Unquiet Mind by Kay Redfield Jamison:

This is a memoir of manic depression/bipolar disorder.

Touched with Fire by Kay Redfield Jamison.

Manic by Terri Cheney:

A memoir of manic depression.

Madness: A Brief History by Roy Porter.

The Day the Voices Stopped by Ken Steele & Claire Berman.

The Motivated Mind by Dr Raj Persaud:

p. 38: Remember goals are worthwhile

The life worth living – if it is about changing and developing yourself to becoming a better human being – must involve goals. If you meet someone without goals then be kind, but you have met someone who is heading for deep unhappiness in the long run, as we feel best about ourselves when we are proud of our achievement in doing something others regard as difficult. All personal pride, self-esteem and self-confidence stem from the realisation of difficult worthwhile goals.

p. 61, para 4: But to change as people we actually need to change our external environment to encourage us to become the kind of person we aspire to.

p. 125, para 6: It was repeatedly found that rewarding people stopped them continuing to do a task when no reward was available. It seemed the external reward changed their motivation from doing a task because they enjoyed it to doing it only for the reward.

p. 127, para 3: The possibility that one could actually reduce the negativity of an activity by combining it with another unpleasant activity is one of the most intriguing results in modern incentive research. This suggests that the best way to engage your six-year-old's interest in reading is to offer her the alternative of doing some boring housework instead!

p. 163, The boss who is a cheat

A very serious but unfortunately not uncommon predicament is when your boss is constantly taking credit for your work. Perhaps he or she let everyone in the last big department meeting think that your new idea was actually their accomplishment. This is the kind of situation that commonly produces fury in doctors, so in a rage they burst into the boss's office and let him or her have a piece of their mind in no uncertain manner.

Although this will make you feel great for a short while – well, until you get back to your clinic – it is not usually conducive to a good long-term relationship with the boss. And remember they usually have more obvious power than you. A motivational analysis of this situation would suggest there are, in fact, only a few reasons why a boss might steal your ideas. First the good news is at least it means they find you a valuable asset to the organization – if only because you come up with good ideas that they can filch.

This kind of boss is usually insecure about their own ability and therefore extremely threatened by talented juniors, so it's absolutely imperative you don't do anything that makes them feel you pose a danger to them. This can lead to an extremely uncomfortable existence ... or a posting to Outer Mongolia. This kind of boss usually responds to a lot of praise for their own work, as they are not used to getting these kinds of strokes, which you should then turn to your advantage. You must, however, protect your own work by presenting ideas you have as formally as possible, preferably at meetings where the proceedings are minuted or in memos that record for posterity who came up with what first.

The best defence against stealing is to have an audience who witness your ideas being presented. This doesn't mean you can't let your boss steal more minor ideas, as this merely encourages their dependence on you. Once they are utterly clingy, turn this to your advantage by requiring more compensation for your assistance in the future. There is no surer path to career advancement than when your boss feels their future is tied up with yours.

p. 222: 'The unlikely fact that doing more gives you greater energy to achieve more is a timeless success secret' Frank Bettger

p. 297 – I tend to be a bit of a work addict.

p. 320, para 3: Consistent anhedonia is a hallmark of depression

p. 379, para 5: The amazing finding suggests that having a smaller hippocampus predisposes you to develop traumatic stress, and may even predict that you will suffer from mental health problems if you are stressed.

Schizophrenia by Max Birchwood & Chris Jackson.

The Bell Jar by Sylvia Plath:

A fictional story about depression which is thought to be a great novel. I think it's quite good.

The Mandarins by Simone de Beauvoir:

This book is set mostly in France in the years after the liberation of France from the Nazis in World War II. The main characters are intellectuals and much of the conversation is about politics and siding with the Russians rather than the Americans. One of the main characters, Anne, is a psychiatrist and another main character is Henri, an author and newspaper editor. Paula's affair with Henri comes to an end and she goes mad (I would say she sounds rather paranoid and may be a paranoid schizophrenic) but Anne does not seem to know what's wrong with her, which suggests to me that Simone de Beauvoir was no expert on psychiatry. Anne herself has an affair in America and when that ends she briefly considers suicide but she decides not to.

This book is very long (the book ends on page 736) and its main themes are love and politics. As far as I can tell it is well written and it sustained my interest so I recommend this book if you are interested in these themes or want to know something of what life was like in France shortly after the occupation. However, mental illness is focussed on in only a very minor part of the book, despite making the top five novels on madness. I give the book 7 out of 10 as a novel.

Cognitive Therapy for Delusions, Voices and Paranoia by Paul Chadwick et al.

Recovery from Schizophrenia by Richard Warner.

Schizophrenia Revealed by Michael Foster Green.

Your Drug May Be Your Problem by Peter R. Breggin & David Cohen:

p. 36, lines 4-9: And the original "antipsychotic" drug, Thorazine, was first used by a French surgeon who noticed that it was useful in making surgical patients indifferent or apathetic toward the pain that they were undergoing. Scientific evidence can be marshalled to support the hypothesis that most psychiatric drugs "work" by producing a kind of anaesthesia of the mind, spirit, or feelings.

p. 77, 2nd to last para: Neuroleptics have their main impact by blunting the highest functions of the brain in the frontal lobes and the closely connected basal ganglia. They can also impair the reticular activating or "energizing" system of the brain. These impairments result in relative degrees of apathy, indifference, emotional blandness, conformity, and submissiveness, as well as a reduction in all verbalisations, including complaints or protests. It is no exaggeration to call this effect a chemical lobotomy.

p. 79, last paragraph: If such high rates for a dangerous and disabling adverse reaction were reported in relation to drugs used in general medicine, such as antibiotics or blood pressure medication, they would probably be removed from the market.

Vulnerable mental patients, by contrast, are purposely exposed to brain-damaging treatments such as electroshock, psychosurgery, and neuroleptics.

p. 81, para 3, last 2 sentences: These drugs subject almost every system of the body to impairment. Research, including a recent study, indicates that these drugs are toxic to cells in general.

p. 82, para 3: The neuroleptics or antipsychotics are extraordinarily dangerous drugs. If they were not highly profitable drugs used to control a rather helpless, stigmatised, or troubling population, often including involuntary patients, these drugs would not be so freely prescribed. They might even be taken off the market.

p. 126, para 4: Coming off drugs – especially strong depressants such as tranquillisers, neuroleptics, or lithium – often involves a potentially dramatic reawakening of the senses. This reawakening can lead to feelings of panic in people who do not realize the extent to which their hearing, touch, taste, or sensations of cold and heat can become unexpectedly acute after having been desensitised or anaesthetized for long periods.

p. 126, para 5, 1st sentence: Withdrawal from several psychiatric drugs – especially central nervous system (CNS) depressants such as tranquillisers, many antidepressants, lithium, and neuroleptics – often provokes bouts of severe insomnia.

p. 163, para 3: A third group of withdrawal reactions involves a wide range of psychological and behavioural symptoms, including insomnia, anxiety, agitation, irritability, and organic psychosis. Psychotic withdrawal symptoms are variously called tardive psychosis, supersensitivity psychosis, or withdrawal psychosis. Frequently accompanied by abnormal movements, they include hallucinations, delusions, confusion, and disorientation.

p. 166, no.3: Neuroleptics should be withdrawn as quickly as possible from patients who have reached forty years of age, since rates for tardive dyskinesia further escalate with age.

p. 166, no.4: Neuroleptic withdrawal should be attempted, if at all possible, in cases where patients who have been taking the drugs for months or years no longer show severe or disabling psychotic symptoms.

p. 167, para 2: Neuroleptics should be completely stopped at the earliest signs of tardive dyskinesia. In the absence of such an emergency, withdrawal from long-term neuroleptics should usually be spread out over at least several months to increase the chances that it will be relatively trouble-free. A 10 percent reduction every two to three months is often warranted. According to the available evidence, the risk of relapse appears greatest between the twelfth and twenty-fourth week after cessation, probably depending on the speed of the withdrawal.

p. 168, para 2, 1st sentence: Based on clinical experience bolstered by research, we suggest that if you are withdrawing from neuroleptics, you should avoid making major changes in your life during and shortly after withdrawal.

The Madness of Adam & Eve – How Schizophrenia Shaped Humanity by David F. Horrobin.

Abnormal Psychology by Philip Kendall/ Constance Hammen.

Beyond Fear by Dorothy Rowe:

Part I: Fear and the Fear of Fear

Greatest? Fear is of annihilation of the self (the meaning structure).

Fear is denied so we are not overwhelmed.

We learn to deny fear and all have psychological problems of some kind to some degree.

We may find bodily 'solutions' in exercise, addictions (e.g., nicotine, alcohol, drugs), eating too much or too little or a lifetime of 'illness'.

Part II: Turning Fear into Madness

The defences we can use against the fear of annihilation are:

1. We can turn fear into (Anxiety) Panics and Phobias. Extraverts are very good at doing this. Fear is more manageable when you give it a name.
2. We can turn fear into Obsessions and Compulsions. Introverts are very good at doing this. An organised world, they believe, should have no room for fear.
3. We can turn fear into Depression. Both extraverts and introverts are good at this. A prison is a safe place.
4. We can turn fear into Mania. Extraverts do this by denying that they are afraid.
5. We can turn fear into Schizophrenia. Introverts are extremely good at doing this.
They escape into their private world.

Part III: Turning Fear into Courage

The way to overcome fear is by holding and helping one another.

Henry's Demons: Living with Schizophrenia, a Father and Son's Story by Patrick and Henry Cockburn:

This interesting autobiography/biography, mainly by a journalist father and a schizophrenic son, tells the story of a young schizophrenic whose illness is particularly bad and fairly unresponsive to treatment. Some parts are written by the schizophrenic and give a clear and vivid account of the thoughts and actions of a psychotic person. The parts by the father and mother I found interesting mostly for what the journalist father had found out about the illness schizophrenia. I think it was quite a good book.

The Shock of the Fall by Nathan Filer is a book about someone who probably has schizophrenia.

Reasons To Stay Alive by Matt Haig:

"Exercise definitely helps me, as does yoga and absorbing myself in something or someone I love, so I keep doing these things."

"Many of the greatest and, well, toughest people of all time have suffered from depression. Politicians, astronauts, poets, painters, philosophers, scientists, mathematicians (a hell of a lot of mathematicians), actors, boxers, peace activists, war leaders, and a billion other people fighting their own battles."

Not Yet Read By Me:

Rowan the Strange by Julie Hearn. This book was on the longlist of the Guardian Children's Fiction prize and is about a teenage boy with schizophrenia in World War II.

Mad Lucas: Strange Story of Victorian England's Most Famous Hermit by Richard Whitmore. This is about James Lucas, who had paranoia and schizophrenia.

Shoot The Damn Dog: A memoir of depression by Sally Brampton. This book was Good Housekeeping Magazine's 'Book of the Month' in February 2008.

How Sadness Survived: The Evolutionary Basis of Depression by Paul Keedwell.

Human Traces by Sebastian Faulks. Rethink's efforts have been reflected in this best-selling book.

Shunned: Discrimination against people with mental illness by Graham Thornicroft.

The boy with the Topknot by Sathnam Sanghera is the story of a British Sikh family's struggle with the father and a daughter having schizophrenia.

Paradoxical Undressing by (Throwing Muses singer) Kristin Hersh is the story of her descent into, and recovery from, schizophrenia.

The heartland: finding and losing schizophrenia by Nathan Filer.

Improving Cognitive Function in the Schizophrenic Patient by RSE Keefe (editor).

Insight and Psychosis: Awareness of Illness in Schizophrenia and Related Disorders, 2nd Edition by Xavier Amador and Anthony David.

There are many books on schizophrenia under the general heading of psychiatry, but it may interest you to know that there are also some under the general area of philosophy.

Chess

I like to think of Schizophrenia, Bipolar Disorder and Depression as being like the King, Queen and Rook pieces in the game of chess. The King is the most seriously important piece, the sine qua non of the game, likewise Schizophrenia is the most serious mental illness generally. Next comes the Queen, with which it is easy to kill/mate the opponent, just as Bipolar Disorder can lead to suicide in many people. Not generally so serious, but potentially deadly is Depression, which can cause death (by suicide) like one can fairly easy kill the opponent with a Rook (and of course King) in chess.

Cognitive Behavioural Therapy

According to National Schizophrenia Fellowship fact sheet 5, 'Cognitive Therapy':

Cognitive Therapy or Cognitive Behavioural Therapy has now been adapted for use with people with schizophrenia. This is a 'talking treatment'.

Cognitive Remediation Therapy

Schizophrenics can have their cognitive impairments ameliorated by Cognitive Remediation Therapy or CRT. Look up 'cognitive remediation therapy' on, e.g., Google Scholar for more information.

Concessionary Schemes that may apply

If you suffer from schizophrenia you may be able to get a bus pass or other travel pass like the *Freedom* pass in London.

Confidence Building

Getting schizophrenia and perhaps depression as well can severely damage your confidence. Confidence building courses may be available at your local mental health unit.

Depression

As a lot of schizophrenics are depressed I thought I would include a section on that.

From *The Guardian*, G2, 20.07.10, p. 14:

Steve Ilardi, a clinical psychologist recommends six things in his "lifestyle based" cure for depression:

1. Be sociable.
2. Engage in meaningful activity.
3. Take regular exercise for 90 minutes a week.
4. Have a diet rich in omega-3 fatty acids (take 1500mg of omega-3 daily with a multivitamin and 500mg vitamin C).
5. 15-30 minutes daily exposure to sunlight/lightbox each morning.
6. Get good quality restorative sleep.

From The Observer, 7.1.18, pages 10-13:

"But between 2011 and 2012, the polling company Gallup conducted the most detailed study ever carried out of how people feel about the thing we spend most of our waking lives doing – our paid work. They found that 13% of people say they are "engaged" in their work – they find it meaningful and look forward to it. Some 63% say they are "not engaged", which is defined as sleepwalking through their workday". And 24% are "actively disengaged": they hate it."

"In its official statement for World Health Day in 2017, the United Nations reviewed the best evidence and concluded that "the dominant biomedical narrative of depression" is based on "biased and selective use of research outcomes" that "must be abandoned". We need to move from "focusing on 'chemical imbalances'", they said, to focusing more on "power imbalances"."

"If you are depressed and anxious, you are not a machine with malfunctioning parts. You are a human being with unmet needs. The only real way out of our epidemic of despair is for all of us, together, to begin to meet those human needs – for deep connection, to the things that really matter in life."

Dietary help for schizophrenics and perhaps others

From *The Observer* 30/5/10 'Fish oil helps schoolchildren to concentrate':

Omega-3 fish oils help people concentrate. Those taking high doses did much better in mathematical challenges... it could also help people with their memory, learning and attention. A lack of DHA has been associated with bipolar disorder and schizophrenia.

From Schizophrenia Digest, Summer 2008, p. 15:

A dietary supplement, N-acetyl cysteine (NAC), available from health food shops, reduces some of the distressing symptoms of schizophrenia not helped by existing medication. In particular, 2g a day of NAC had a significant reduction in negative symptoms, such as loss of motivation, drive, and initiative, and social withdrawal.

About 50% of people diagnosed with schizophrenia do not understand they are ill.

From a Rethink leaflet:

75% of employers say that it would be difficult or impossible to employ someone with schizophrenia. However, 58% of people with schizophrenia can work if supported through Individual Placements and workplace support.

The book *GAPS Gut and Psychology Syndrome: Natural treatment for Autism, Dyspraxia, A.D.D, Dyslexia, A.D.H.D, Depression and Schizophrenia (Revised and Expanded Edition)* By Dr Natasha Campbell-McBride may be helpful. It mentions that schizophrenia did not exist in some South Pacific cultures before grain was introduced.

Dose-Response Curve for Me (Estimated)

Response = (TANH((Dose-250)/40)+1)/2.

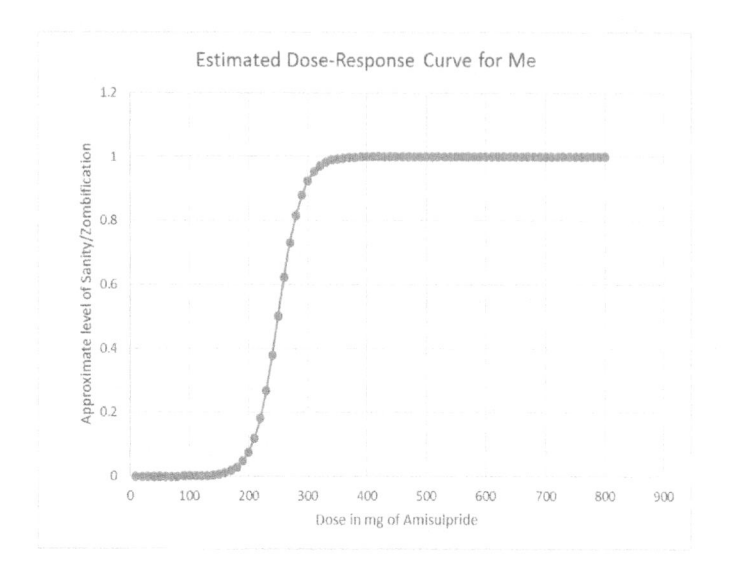

Estimated Dose-Response Curve for Me

(y-axis: Approximate level of Sanity/Zombification; x-axis: Dose in mg of Amisulpride)

There are six daily dosages I would like to talk about that I have tried:

1. 400mg. I was on this first dose for years, and I would describe myself then as mentally dull, sane but inactive regarding proper 'work'- virtually no maths research, instead writing occasional poems and reading popular science.

2. 300mg. I was on this fourth dose (following months on each of 350mg and 325mg) for several years. I would describe myself on this dose as being sane, moderately dull, and fairly inactive regarding proper 'work' – writing books, poems, doing occasional maths research and reading popular science.

3. 275mg. I was on this fifth dose for 46 days. I would describe myself on this dose as sane, active regarding proper work – doing some proper mathematical research, but not sleeping.

4. 287.5mg. I was on this sixth dose for over 2 years. I would describe myself as sane and moderately active regarding proper work – mostly doing mathematical research, reading maths textbooks and writing the occasional poem.

5. 281.25mg. I was on this seventh dose for 67 days. During this time I was sane and active mathematically. The main problem was not getting enough sleep. Hence the move to the next slightly higher dose.

6. 283.33mg. I have been on this eighth dose for nearly 2 years. During this time I have been very active mathematically, producing lots of mathematical output written up properly, and been fairly sane. The main problem with my wellbeing was dealing with a problematic mathematical collaborator who upset me very greatly indeed. Until he upset me things were going very well, and I have managed to continue functioning well since then, considering how much he upset me. Note that there is a book titled "The Toxic University" as well as one titled "Toxic Psychiatry"!

Note that my estimated dose-response curve (which might be shifted and/or stretched horizontally for other schizophrenics) suggests that at some doses a relatively large reduction can be made with little effect, whereas in the more critical region in the 'middle' a very small change in dose can have a big effect.

Famous Schizophrenics

There is a list of famous people with schizophrenia, currently 85 long, with a webpage on each accessible at http://en.wikipedia.org/wiki/List_of_people_with_schizophrenia .

A great artist who developed schizophrenia was Louis Wain (1860-1939). His art changed and became more abstract after getting schizophrenia, but it is all beautiful work to see.

A popular musician with schizophrenia who received great acclaim was Syd Barrett of Pink Floyd.

Donald Campbell, brother of the famous political aide Alistair Campbell, had schizophrenia. There is a fine article about him, by Alistair Campbell in The Sunday Times, 14.8.16, pages 25-26.

Similarly, there is a (much longer) list of famous people with bipolar disorder at

http://en.wikipedia.org/wiki/List_of_people_with_bipolar_disorder .

Films

(See www.imdb.com for more details of the films)

Family Life (1971) – a film that deals with the treatment of a 19-year-old girl for schizophrenia. Based on the TV play *In Two Minds* by David Mercer.

A Beautiful Mind (2001) – A film about the real-life schizophrenic mathematician John Nash who wins a Nobel Prize for his work. See also http://www.pbs.org/wgbh/amex/nash/ .

Drummer Boy (2002) – A film mentioned in Schizophrenia Digest, Fall 2003, p.31.

People Say I'm Crazy (2003) – A documentary mentioned in Schizophrenia Digest, Fall 2003, p.31.

Out of the Shadow (2004) – Documentary about the film-maker's mother and her battle with schizophrenia. Featured in Schizophrenia Digest, Winter 2006.

Proof (2005) – A film about a daughter of a schizophrenic mathematician.

Shine (1996) – This is a film about a brilliant young pianist who has a breakdown but eventually recovers to some extent.

The Soloist (2009):

The Soloist stars Robert Downey Jr as newspaper reporter Steve Lopez who, whilst looking for a story, notices a violinist Nathaniel Ayers playing a violin with just two strings remaining by Beethoven's Statue in Los Angeles. He introduces himself and over time they get to know each other a little. It turns out Nathaniel is a talented musician who attended the Juilliard Music Academy and Steve tries to get Nathaniel to move into a flat rather than living on the street. Nathaniel is encouraged by Steve to attend a place called LAMPS where mentally ill people spend some time and, eventually, he gets reunited with his sister. An attempt to get Nathaniel to give a recital ends in disaster with Nathaniel running out at the start. Also, Nathaniel is violent towards Steve when Steve tries to get Nathaniel to sign papers saying he has a schizophrenic mind in order to get his flat, but in the end they become friends again and Nathaniel stays in the flat. At the end of the movie Steve, Nathaniel, Nathaniel's sister and Steve's ex-wife are shown attending a classical music concert together.

That is the extent of the improvement in the situation of Nathaniel and it is stated that his mental state is no better than when Steve first met him (he doesn't take medication), but he has a friend in Steve and is in touch with his sister, which Steve believes helps. This film is based on a true story and is a bit like both A Beautiful Mind and Shine, and is nearly as good. I was made aware of the movie by the excellent upbeat magazine Schizophrenia Digest, which sadly seems to have been discontinued.

Me, Myself & Irene (2000):

I bought a DVD of this film because I had previously discovered on a website that this film featured schizophrenia and was curious about it. In this comedy, the main character Charlie, played by Jim Carrey, is a policeman in Rhode Island who is left by his wife shortly after getting married, she having met a very short black guy who is a leading member of Mensa. (She is also a leading member of Mensa). Charlie doesn't really react to the loss of his wife except by becoming too nice and accommodating to be a good policeman and repressing his tough side. Many years later his tough side comes out in the form of a hyper-aggressive alter ego, Hank, and Hank and Charlie battle it out for control of their common body and the affections of Irene (played by Renee Zellweger). Eventually Charlie integrates his nice and tough sides and wins over Irene.

Charlie/Hank is described in the movie as both a schizophrenic and also as having a split personality disorder so this film confuses schizophrenia with multiple personality disorder. I did not find it irredeemably bad, though my mother described it as appalling (it being unnecessarily crude), and it may harm or reinforce people's (mis)conception of schizophrenia. It's probably not a film that would appeal to Mensa members or people who know about schizophrenia, even though it features both.

Spider (2002):

Spider stars Ralph Fiennes as a man called Spider who arrives at some kind of hostel/group home for people with mental illness and keeps thinking about his past. He wears four shirts on top of each other and there is an amusing remark from a fellow mentally ill person in the home who says "Clothes maketh the man. The less substantial the man, the more clothes are needed" or words to that effect. Spider is very quiet and mumbles to himself and scribbles notes that are incomprehensible in a notebook. He remembers how his father had killed his mother and she had been replaced by a "cheap tart" and how he had rigged up some string to their gas oven and gassed to death the cheap tart. At the same time as recalling this Spider comes to think the woman who runs the group home is the tart from his childhood grown older and he becomes paranoid and steals her keys and takes a hammer and it seems is just about to kill her when he realises she is not the tart after all. He was clearly having a delusion/hallucination just as he falsely believed his mother had been replaced by the tart in his childhood. He does not kill the hostel keeper unlike when he killed his mother in his childhood, but, now as well as then he is taken to the Asylum.

This is a bleak tale and, although much praised in the Radio Times, I do not think it helps the cause of schizophrenics at all, portraying them as murderers or potential murderers and people to be frightened of. The film is based on a book but I don't know if the book was fact or fiction.

Also involving schizophrenia, but not seen by me yet:

The Story of Ruth (1981) – starring Connie Booth, who also appeared in a stage version.

Keane (2004)

Canvas (2006) – starring Marcia Gay Harden, Joe Pantoliano and Devon Gearhart.

Food supplements for schizophrenics

The Schizophrenia Association of Great Britain used to issue a nutrient pack which was generally considered helpful for schizophrenics. The recommended daily doses were:

High Potency Fish Oil: up to 3 capsules

Vitamin B12: 1000ug

Folic Acid: 400ug

Vitamin B1: 100mg

Vitamin C: 1 or 2 times 1000mg

Vitamin B Complex: 1 tablet. Contains B1 (100mg), B2 (100mg), B3 (100mg), B6 (100mg), Folic acid (100ug), B12 (100ug), Biotin (100ug), Pantothenic acid (100mg), Choline (100mg), Inositol (100mg), PABA (30mg)

Magnesium: 1 to 3 times 150mg

Selenium plus vitamins: 1 tablet. Contains Selenium 200ug, Vitamin A (450ug), Vitamin C (90mg), Vitamin E (30mg)

Vitamin D3: 1000IU.

A book I have used to guide me in what supplements to take for schizophrenia is Optimum Nutrition for the Mind by Patrick Holford.

A book has been written recommending Turmeric for schizophrenia: Turmeric Curcumin For Schizophrenia: All you need to know on how turmeric curcumin treats schizophrenia by Dr Sylvester John.

General Mental Health

From The Sun, 3.11.15, page 2, Why your body needs an MOT: "Our exclusive survey on men's health also found that half of the nation's fellas have experienced a mental health issue."

Group Homes

I have visited three homes for people with mental illness, and they all seemed well kept and the staff seemed pleasant.

Half-Life of Anti-psychotic Medication

Half-life	Anti-psychotic
3-20 hours	Risperidone
4-9 hours	Prochlorperazine
6-10 hours	Benperidol
6-26 hours	Clozapine
7-12 hours	Quetiapine
About 8 hours	Sulpiride
About 12 hours	Amisulpride
About 12 hours	Pericyazine
20-40 hours	Lurasidone
20-40 hours	Promazine
21-24 hours	Haloperidol
About 22 hours	Trifluoperazine
About 23 hours	Paliperidone
About 24 hours	Asenapine
About 24 hours	Zuclopenthixol dihydrochloride
About 30 hours	Chlorpromazine
About 30 hours	Levomepromazine

31-52 hours	Olanzapine
About 35 hours	Flupentixol
55-150 hours	Pimozide
75-146 hours	Aripiprazole
2-8 days	Cariprazine
3-6 days	Risperidone (depot)
17-112 days	Fluphenazine decanoate
17-21 days	Flupentixol decanoate
About 19 days	Zuclopenthixol
About 19 days	Zuclopenthixol decanoate
About 21 days	Haloperidol decanoate
25-139 days	Paliperidone palmitate
29-46 days	Aripiprazole (depot)
About 30 days	Olanzapine pamoate monohydrate

Heartland

Apparently, schizophrenia used to be known as the "heartland" of psychiatry.

Influence on weight of various drugs

Source unknown.

Drug class	Drugs causing weight gain	weight loss	Drugs thought not to affect weight
Antidepressants	Amitriptyline	Fluoxetine	SSRIs
	Imipramine, other TCAs	?Bupropion	Moclobemide
	Isocarboxazid		Venlafaxine
	Phenelzine		Trazodone
	?Tranylcypromine		Nefazodone
			Amoxapine
Antipsychotics	Phenothiazines	None	Molindone (not available in UK)
	Depot preparations		Loxapine
	Haloperidol		?Perphenazine
	Clozapine		Ziprasidone (not licensed in UK at time of publication)
	Olanzapine		
	Quetiapine		
	Risperidone		
	Zotepine		
Anxiolytics	None	None	Benzodiazepines
Mood stabilisers /antiepileptic Drugs	Lithium	Topiramate	Lamotrigine
	Sodium Valproate	Felbamate	Gabapentin
	Vigabatrin		Phenobarbitone
	?Carbamazepine		Phenytoin
Stimulants	None	Amphetamines	?Modafanil
		Methylphenidate	

Information from the World Wide Web

www.comingoff.com (Coming off Psychiatric Medication – a site that is no more):

On Atypical anti-psychotics:

Individuals who had no psychiatric history have been given a course of neuroleptic treatment, and when the neuroleptics were abruptly withdrawn some of these individuals developed 'psychotic' symptoms.

James Middleton

James Middleton, the brother of Katherine Middleton who is the Duchess of Cambridge, has suffered from depression. Perhaps this and the Duke and Duchess of Cambridge being interested in and speaking about mental health might help matters for schizophrenics a little.

Links between Schizophrenia, Autism and Bipolar Disorder

From The Sun 12.2.18, page 15, article titled: *"Gene link to autism"*: "Autism, schizophrenia and bipolar disorder are all caused by the same gene mutations in the brain, research suggests. The three major psychiatric conditions share similar variations in RNA, a substance which works alongside DNA. Study chief Prof Daniel Geschwind of the University of California says the test findings are "a large step forward" in understanding the causes of mental illness and could lead to better treatments." (More details in *Scientific American*.)

From The Observer, 17.11.19, page 22, article titled: *"Mutating genes feed persistence of schizophrenia"*: "In particular, gene mutations that affect brain cell synapses and the developing brain appear to have a strong effect in leading to cases of schizophrenia, and also other psychological conditions, including autism and bipolar disorder."

Medication Side Effects

The following website is a place where you can report suspected side effects of medication. https://yellowcard.mhra.gov.uk .

From SZ Magazine, Winter 2010:

'Numerous studies have indicated that Abilify has the advantage of causing fewer long-term side effects, such as lower weight gain and less increase in cholesterol.' – so it would seem that most anti-psychotics increase cholesterol! ☹

From Schizophrenia Digest, Fall 2008, p. 27:

"... there are several things that can be done to overcome sedative side effects:

1. Take all of your medicine in the evening about 1-2 hours before you plan to retire to bed – that way the sleepiness from the medications will help you sleep and should wear off by the time you awaken
2. Discuss with your doctor trying a lower dose of your medication.

A new antipsychotic, aripiprazole (Abilify) is the only medication for psychosis that does not affect prolactin levels, so your doctor may switch you to this medication if your periods have stopped.

Mind Leaflets

The organization Mind has many useful leaflets, such as *How to cope with sleep problems*, *Making sense of antipsychotics*, *Understanding schizophrenia*, *How to deal with anger*, *How to support someone who feels suicidal* and *How to cope with student life*.

Mystery Shoppers

Some NHS Trusts may allow patients to be a 'Mystery Shopper' and report back on how they are treated by receptionists and psychiatrists when having outpatient appointments.

Notorious Treatment of Schizophrenics in Nazi Germany

From TV:

The schizophrenics were gassed in Nazi Germany as a trial run of methods of killing prior to killing millions of Jews.

Notorious treatment of the mentally ill in the past and present even in the UK and US!

Lobotomies

Many patients, including schizophrenics, were given a Lobotomy. This deliberately damaged the brain and left some patients as cabbages or even dead.

The book *My Lobotomy: A Memoir* by Howard Dully and Charles Fleming tells one patient's tale.

I find it greatly cheering to note that the man who invented it, who was misguidedly given a Nobel Prize for it, was shot by one of his patients! ☺

From The Daily Mirror Wednesday 15.04.09, 'Unfit for a Dog', p. 17:

A farmer with schizophrenia was taken advantage of by a cruel couple and swindled out of his money and died of scurvy after being made to live in a barn.

Notorious treatment of troublesome citizens as if mentally ill

In the Soviet Union, political dissidents were put in mental asylums.

From The Guardian, date unknown:

'Chinese petitioners forced into mental asylums, claims report':

18 people claim that they have been force-fed psychiatric drugs and held in mental hospitals in China.

Opportunities to be a service-user researcher/service user expert

From The Guardian, Tuesday 25/8/09:

There are service-user researchers at Lancaster University's Spectrum centre for mental health research, St George's, University of London, and the Service User Research Enterprise team at the Institute of Psychiatry, King's College, University of London.

Sometimes The Royal College of Psychiatrists Research Unit (www.rcpsych.ac.uk) wants service user experts to do a small amount of work for them and will pay for it.

You can earn some money from an 'Experts by Experience' group like the one at the University of Bedfordshire.

Optimizing Schizophrenia

Unfortunately, psychiatrists don't seem to have great hopes or aspirations for their schizophrenic patients. In my 'care plan' from 2002 it stated as the Goal/Objective: "For [his] mental state to be maintained so he can function adequately in the community." Also, once a dosage of a drug is found that works reasonably well, that dose is generally stuck to, even though the patient might function much better on a lower dose. Just a couple of years ago a psychiatrist told me that "once a dose is found that works, they keep to that dose" or words to that effect. As an example of what often happens, here is a quote from *Perceptions*, Summer 2013, issue 42, p. 5: "There, at 18 years of age my hefty initial schizophrenic medication, i.e., depixol depot injections – resulted in severely debilitating side effects – like Parkinsonism and being constantly over sedated. In other words, "society" drugged me up and left me to rot. OK!"

Reductions in dose that are attempted are normally too large (say 50% or 25%), resulting in 'failure' at the lower dose and a resigned return to the old dose, whereas improvements in functioning could be achieved through a reduction by no more than about 10% and perhaps as little as 1%. I think many schizophrenics could function much better than they do by finding, through a series of small adjustments, the *optimal* dose of a helpful medication. Dosages should not be confined to whole numbers of tablets but rather fractions with small denominators should be considered, and decreases or increases in dose by as little as 1% could be made beneficially – see the section of this book titled *Dose-Response Curve For Me (Estimated)* – until an optimal dose is converged upon, possibly using the method of *binary search* once a dose that is too low and another that is too high has been discovered, as implemented in the following algorithm.

An Algorithm For Finding The Optimal Dose

Starting With A Dose On Which The Schizophrenic Does Well

1. Choose a convenient new dose that is less than the current dose but at least 90% of the current dose and switch to that dose.
2. If doing well* on the new dose (e.g., adequate sleep, eating alright, sane) then after a period of at least a further 3 months go to Step 1.
3. If not doing well* on the new dose (e.g., inadequate sleep, not eating alright, precarious or lost sanity) then choose a new dose that is a convenient dose as close to the average of the current dose and the old dose as possible, and switch to that dose at the next medication time.
4. Decide if doing well or not* on the current dose. If doing well, continue on the current dose for at least another 3 months, otherwise go at the next medication time to Step 5.
5. If possible (i.e., the change in dose is not too small or would result in too little sleep), choose a new convenient dose that is equal to, or as close as possible on one side of, (and closer than the current dose is to) the average of the highest dose on which not doing well and the lowest dose on which doing well. Otherwise go to Step 7.
6. Switch to the new dose and go to Step 4.

7. Continue indefinitely at the lowest dose that kept the schizophrenic doing well.

   * This will probably take weeks or months to decide, even with a medication with a short half-life like the amisulpride which I am taking.

A flowchart summarizing this algorithm is displayed on the next page.

The idea of optimizing the dose of antipsychotic medication might be fruitfully extended to sufferers of psychoses other than schizophrenia who are given antipsychotics to take, and indeed might be applied to other psychiatric drugs in the opinion of the author. However, as stated in the preface, please consult a psychiatrist before altering a dose of such a medication.

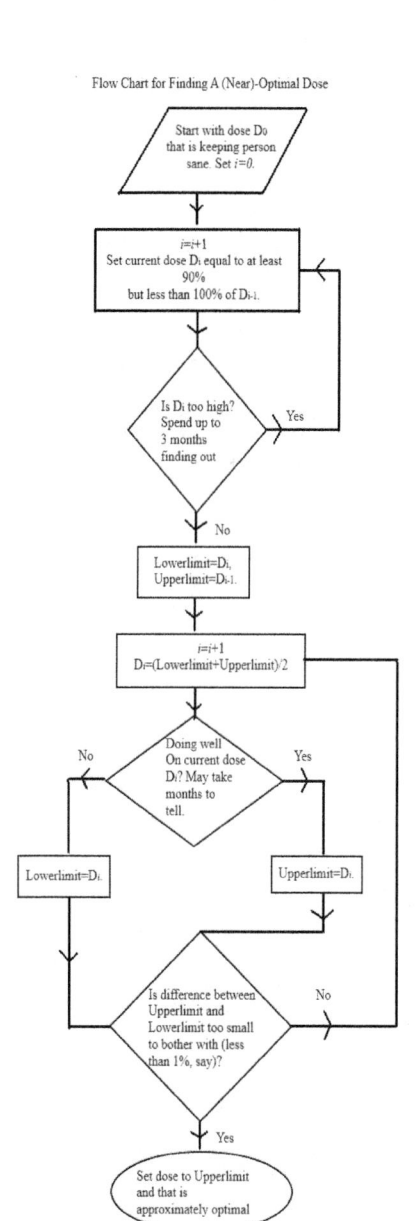

Flow Chart for Finding A (Near)-Optimal Dose

```
            ┌──────────────────────┐
            │ Start with dose D₀   │
            │ that is keeping person│
            │ sane. Set i=0.       │
            └──────────┬───────────┘
                       ▼
            ┌──────────────────────┐
            │       i=i+1          │◄──────┐
            │ Set current dose Dᵢ  │       │
            │ equal to at least 90%│       │
            │ but less than 100%   │       │
            │ of Dᵢ₋₁.             │       │
            └──────────┬───────────┘       │
                       ▼                    │
                  ╱─────────╲               │
                 ╱ Is Dᵢ too ╲   Yes        │
                ╱  high?     ╲──────────────┘
                ╲ Spend up to╱
                 ╲ 3 months ╱
                  ╲finding  ╱
                   ╲  out  ╱
                    ╲─┬──╱
                      │ No
                      ▼
            ┌──────────────────────┐
            │ Lowerlimit=Dᵢ,       │
            │ Upperlimit=Dᵢ₋₁.     │
            └──────────┬───────────┘
                       ▼
            ┌──────────────────────┐
            │       i=i+1          │◄────────┐
            │ Dᵢ=(Lowerlimit+      │         │
            │    Upperlimit)/2     │         │
            └──────────┬───────────┘         │
                       ▼                      │
                  ╱─────────╲                 │
         No      ╱ Doing well╲      Yes       │
     ┌─────────╱ On current  ╲─────────┐     │
     │         ╲ dose Dᵢ?    ╱          │     │
     │          ╲ May take  ╱           │     │
     │           ╲months to╱            │     │
     │            ╲ tell. ╱             │     │
     │             ╲─────╱              │     │
     ▼                                  ▼     │
┌──────────────┐              ┌──────────────┐│
│Lowerlimit=Dᵢ.│              │Upperlimit=Dᵢ.││
└──────┬───────┘              └──────┬───────┘│
       │                              │        │
       └──────────────┬───────────────┘        │
                      ▼                         │
                 ╱─────────╲                    │
                ╱ Is diff.  ╲      No           │
               ╱ between     ╲──────────────────┘
               ╲Upperlimit & ╱
                ╲Lowerlimit ╱
                 ╲too small╱
                  ╲(<1%)? ╱
                   ╲─┬──╱
                     │ Yes
                     ▼
            ╭──────────────────────╮
            │ Set dose to Upperlimit│
            │ and that is           │
            │ approximately optimal │
            ╰──────────────────────╯
```

Organizations

Though now shut down, there used to be *The Schizophrenia Association of Great Britain (SAGB)*, web: www.sagb.co.uk

Rethink:

Rethink is the operating name of National Schizophrenia Fellowship. Their strapline is 'We improve the lives of people severely affected by mental illness through our network of local groups and services, expert information and successful campaigning. Our goal is to make sure everyone affected by severe mental illness has a good quality of life.'

Web Address:

www.rethink.org .

Mind:

This organization has lots of clubhouses where those with mental illness can socialise and do various activities. Also, they have produced relevant publications, such as the leaflet *Understanding Schizophrenia*. Local Mind branches sometimes offer a Healthy Aspirations course, and courses such as Personal Wellbeing and Mental Health Awareness, Confidence Building, Goal Planning and Cognitive Behavioural Therapy (CBT).

Web: www.mind.org.uk

Ace Enterprises (ELFT)

Community-based mental health services providing meaningful activity, group sessions and training for adults of working age.

Tel 01582 708200.

ACE stands for Alternative Choices into Employment.

Time To Change:

Time to Change is a campaign to end mental health discrimination. Their website is

www.time-to-change.org.uk and they have produced adverts on TV and have published articles in, e.g., *The Daily Mirror*.

Time to Change is on Facebook (see https://www.facebook.com/timetochange)

The Shaw Trust:

They help people with health problems get back into employment. Their website is https://www.shawtrust.org.uk/ .

Impact MH: Mental Health Peer Support

Website: https://www.impactmh.org.uk , telephone 01582 797596.

They used to run a course called Peer Support Programme.

A previous group asking for service user views was called *Whole Life, Whole Systems*.

SANE (Schizophrenia A National Emergency):

Web address: www.sane.org.uk.

British Psychological Society:

You can find a psychologist near you at http://www.bps.org.uk/.

Richmond Fellowship:

Richmond Fellowship is a national mental health charity. It says on their website: "Supporting people with mental ill health on their recovery journeys for 60 years" Their web address is www.richmondfellowship.org.uk.

Campaign Against Living Miserably (CALM):

The Campaign Against Living Miserably is leading a movement against suicide, the single biggest killer of men under 45 in the UK and the cause of 18 deaths every day. Their website is at www.thecalmzone.net.

Relevant information: www.stopsuicidepledge.org/ and Samaritans: 08457 90 90 90 (24-hour national helpline).

togetherall

The website https://togetherall.com/en-gb/ says it is a safe online community where people support each other anonymously to improve mental health and wellbeing.

Hub Of Hope

The website, www.hubofhope.co.uk, seems to consist mainly of a database of mental health support available in the UK.

Samaritans

Their website is www.samaritans.org and their telephone number 116 123. They support anyone who needs help in the UK and Republic of Ireland.

The Consortium for Therapeutic Communities

This has a website www.therapeuticcommunities.org.

National Women and Mental Health Information Line has a telephone number – 0845 300 0911.

Support Line has a website www.supportline.org.uk.

The Mental Health Foundation has a website www.mentalhealth.org.uk.

Penrose

Penrose caters for those with mental health problems and features on the website: https://socialinterestgroup.org.uk/.

The British Red Cross now offers help for loneliness, see, e.g., www.Redcross.org.uk/tackleloneliness.

Other uses of drugs used for schizophrenia

From www.medicalnewstoday.com , news article 10 October 2006:

The U.S. Food and Drug Administration (FDA) today approved a new use of one of the leading prescription antipsychotic medications, Risperdal(R) (risperidone), for the treatment of *irritability associated with autistic disorder*, including symptoms of aggression, deliberate self-injury, temper tantrums, and quickly changing moods, in children and adolescents aged 5 to 16 years.

From The Guardian, Tuesday April 1st 2008:

'Warning on drugs for Alzheimer's patients in nursing homes':

The "chemical cosh" antipsychotic drugs that are widely prescribed for people with Alzheimer's disease in nursing homes do more harm than good, according to a study published today. ....The study ....found that long-term use of the drugs led to a significant deterioration in the thinking and verbal skills of patients.

From File on 4, BBC Radio 4, 17.06.08:

One elderly person was a chatterbox and 'with it' but after being given quetiapine was over-sedated, zombie-like and suffered drowsiness, low blood pressure and fainting. There are 9 atypical psychotics in common use. These cause an increased risk of stroke, chest infection, pneumonia, risk of death. Doctors give 0% to 90% of dementia patients these drugs. They are being prescribed to keep people quiet (because of over-worked staff). If given Olanzapine they become unusually drowsy and sleeping all the time.

From The Observer 20.04.08, 'Under the 'chemical cosh'':

Years ago I was admitted to hospital with anorexia. The drug I was bullied into swallowing was Largactil, whose nickname is 'liquid cosh'. It stupefied me. I could not follow the simplest newspaper article. They sent me back to work, still dosed up, with a supply of pills to take at lunchtime. I was too exhausted to carry out the easiest task and constantly fell asleep at my desk. It was horribly humiliating.

Now I see that psychiatrists are robbing Alzheimer's patients of what is left of their capacity to think by forcing drugs in them, just to shut them up and make life easy for the staff. This is abuse and a violation of patients' human rights.

Name and address supplied.

From the web:

Neuroleptics are the most consistently useful medications for tic suppression in people with Tourette's Syndrome. The most common side effects of neuroleptics include sedation, weight gain, and cognitive dulling.

Also in the context of Tourette's syndrome, adverse effects mentioned are:

Motor: drug-induced parkinsonism, akinesia, akathisia, acute dystonia, tardive dyskinesia, oculogyric crisis, extrapyramidal reactions, restlessness; CNS: sedation, drowsiness, decrease in cognitive function, anxiety; Autonomic: dry eyes/mouth, urinary retention, diaphoresis, hypersalivation; GI: increased appetite, weight gain, anorexia, constipation, hepatitis; Other: dysphoria, social and school phobias, heatstroke, polydipsia, impotence, photosensitivity, rashes, galactorrhea, hyperpyrexia, anaemia, leukopenia.

Alas, some GPs have prescribed anti-psychotics for tinnitus. I briefly suffered from a high-pitched noise in one ear and was prescribed with *stemetil*, an anti-psychotic, which I took initially as I trusted the GP, dropped after a day or two after reading the leaflet that came with the tablets, and which may have seeded my psychological troubles six years later! ☹

Personal Note

16.11.15 Discovered from the internet that high prolactin (caused by my medication) leads to less hormone responsible for the normal functioning of the testicles and therefore presumably less testosterone and hence less maintenance or development of muscles mass and so weakness in muscles. However, recent weight training with dumbbells suggests I can build strength and so counter one effect of the medication.

Photography

Big Brother by Louis Quail is a book of photographs of his brother (who has paranoid schizophrenia) and his brother's girlfriend.

Plays

From *Building a Healthier Britain* (BBC Radio4, 2005):

The play called *Blue/Orange* by Joe Penhall is about a young mental patient and the doctors treating him and has won awards. (See, e.g., http://www.bbc.co.uk/programmes/b0074r35 for more information).

From The Guardian, Tuesday May 1st 2007, p. 36:

Elling, A new version by Simon Bent, based on the novel by Ingvar Ambjornsen is about two psychiatric patients trying to make a life in the community.

From The Observer, 21.02.10, page 11:

There is a play called *Calico* by Michael Hastings about the relationship between James Joyce's schizophrenic daughter Lucia and the young Samuel Beckett.

Bedlam is a play by Nell Leyshon set in an asylum. She has won the 2005 Evening Standard Most Promising Playwright Award.

Prejudice in the Workplace

From an article by Denis Campbell, Health Policy Editor, in a newspaper article dated some time in 2015 or afterwards: "few people believe that a person with depression (17%) or schizophrenia (8%) that is well controlled by medication would be as likely as others to be promoted. And about one in three think that the medical history of someone with either condition should make a difference to their chances of gaining promotion."

Problems which are more likely to arise in children of schizophrenics

From The Guardian, date unknown, 'Autism's link to mental illness in parents':

"Our research shows that mothers and fathers diagnosed with schizophrenia were about twice as likely to have a child diagnosed with autism."

Psychoeducation

You might be fortunate enough to be offered a place in a psychoeducation group by your local mental hospital where you learn about mental illnesses including your own. Of course, this book is like an education in schizophrenia and to a lesser extent depression and manic depression.

Psychosis

There are several types of psychosis, of which schizophrenia is just one. The full list given to me in my psychoeducation at Calnwood Court, Luton is as follows.

Drug-induced psychosis

Organic Psychosis

Brief Reactive Psychosis

Delusional Disorder

Schizophrenia

Schizophreniform Disorder

Bipolar Disorder

Schizoaffective Disorder

Psychotic Depression

Publications for schizophrenics and others

Perceptions:

The quarterly magazine *Perceptions* of the National Perceptions Forum (a service user/survivor run organization) is entertaining and informing, containing cartoons, poems, letters and articles by service users. Their website is www.voicesforum.org . The magazine comes free with Perceptions membership, which is free.

SZ Magazine (formerly called Schizophrenia Digest):

This used to be an excellent quarterly magazine published in the USA and Canada. It included letters, articles, news on schizophrenia-related matters, research updates and physical health matters relevant to schizophrenics. Its website was www.szmagazine.com and this contained, amongst other things, the excellent 'Conversations with Bill MacPhee'.

Publishers Dealing With Mental Health Topics

Chipmunkapublishing (web: www.chipmunkapublishing.co.uk) specialises in mental health books, including lots of personal stories/memoirs.

Radio Programmes on Madness

A good programme on BBC Radio 4 is *All in the Mind.*

Another source is www.madnessradio.net .

Reducing Medication

Medication should only be reduced very gradually and slowly. See, e.g., the book *Your Drug May Be Your Problem* under books in this publication. As an illustration of this here is my medication reduction diary.

Medication Reduction Diary:

My normal dose of antipsychotic, amisulpride, is 200mg in the morning, 200mg at night which I have been on continuously for 4.5 years. Following the psychiatrist's suggestion that I reduced the dose to 100mg in the morning and 200mg at night, I decided to be more cautious and chose to take 150mg in the morning and 200mg at night. For the next 16 days I recorded how I was.

Day 1 (Wednesday 28/02/07)

Felt less lethargic walking down to Befrienders than usual, but surely not due to the change in dose – too early for that, maybe psychological only. Other than that, I feel quite normal.

Day 2

Unusually depressed in morning before got up – think due to thinking about cognitive impairment. Tune to Steptoe & Son came into my head – haven't had that happen before. Went to drop-in at Befrienders & was slightly miffed when person I spoke to (new person) said little back to me. Reconciled myself to it after a while, but don't normally get this miffed.

Back home Dad spoke to me and perhaps I was more irritated and tetchy than on old dose.

Day 3

Woke up early - 5:49 am and did not want more sleep. Had an erection without wanting to go to toilet (usually want to go to toilet) so that's an improvement sexually. Felt normal at Befrienders, maybe even quite good. Had fruit tea (suspect was flavoured Green Tea, left in my mug stewing for a long time by mistake). Went to bed at 9 pm.

Day 4

Woke up at 11:15 pm at night after only 2 hrs sleep. Felt a bit unwell (felt sick) and alert. Vomited (3 heaves) at 1:15 am. During the day felt exhausted but fairly wide-awake and only slept a very little. Went to bed at 7:30 pm.

Day 5

Had quite a lot of sleep between going to bed and getting up at 8 am – maybe 8 hours (though woke up a few times). Feel a lot better than yesterday. However, still very physically tired, though mentally quite alert and awake. Went to bed at 9 pm.

Day 6

No sleep (except perhaps between about 4 and 7 am). Feeling very tired physically - exhausted really. At 1 pm vomited 6 times. Had a quiet day. Went to bed at 7:30 pm.

Day 7

Had maybe 10-12 hours sleep. Feel mentally alert and awake. Felt like doing something to stop self being bored (do not usually feel so keen on activity), so downloaded emails (840) and paid credit card bill and membership fee for running club. Feeling more of a mental appetite for doing things – is it my empty stomach or optimism or reduced dose of amisulpride? Went to bed soon after 10 pm.

Day 8

Woke up at 5:24 am, rested/slept a tiny bit till 7:15 am. Ate breakfast and small lunch. Felt a bit fearful and depressed in afternoon on bed, but felt a bit better later. Went to bed at 9:30 pm.

Day 9

Woke up at 3:30 am to go to toilet. Had some more sleep (maybe hours) till 8:30 am when got up. Had a reasonably active day – no doze in afternoon and went to bed at 11 pm.

Day 10

Woke up 2 or 3 times in night, on last occasion had an erection without wanting to go to toilet. Had about 6 hrs sleep and then awake for a short while then dozed/slept till 8:30 am (did not hear 8 am alarm). Went to hospital, had blood test on my own and had a 2-hour sleep after lunch. Stools were very much lighter than usual – light brown in evening. Went to bed at 9:30 pm.

Day 11

Woke up at 6:30 am and again at 8:30 am. Had an ejaculation. Went for a 3-mile walk even though felt physically tired. Whilst I may be more awake and a bit livelier on 350mg, I still don't have as much to say for myself as I would like. Had a reasonable day and evening (including visit by B). Had more mental energy than physical today, feeling a bit tired physically in afternoon. Went to bed at 10:30 pm.

Day 12

Woke up about 7:52 am (so about 9.5 hours sleep). Still a bit physically tired. Went for a 3-mile walk in afternoon and had a doze afterwards. Did some reading and watching TV. Went to bed at 10:40 pm.

Day 13

Got up at 9 am, having slept nearly all the time since going to bed. Maybe slightly less tired physically than on previous days. Back almost entirely to eating and drinking normally (though haven't tried new herbal tea yet). Walked to town and back 3 times (played pool, went to Befrienders and got tablets). Went to bed at 10:30 pm.

Day 14

Woke up at 5:20 am and later at 6:20 am and finally got up at 8:13 am. Had a small ejaculation. Went to see psychiatrist (no change in meds, next appointment June) and had a doze after got home. Was a bit depressed following meeting and so dozed after lunch. Then had an ayurvedic tea, as I thought I'm back to normal stomach-wise. Also, I think I'm back to how I was on 400mg mentally – no livelier mentally. Went for a 3-mile walk. Went to bed at 11 pm.

Day 15

Woke up at 6:30 am, dozed till 8:50 am then got up. Stools looked normal medium – dark brown colour (darker than during recent days and back to old normal on 400mg). Did art at Befrienders, snooker at Racks (back to normal Wednesday activities). Went to bed at 11:40 pm.

Day 16

Woke up at 7:20 am, slept again till 10 am when got up. Weighed 11st 3.5lbs so still at least 8lbs lighter than on Day 0 and same as after sickness. Stools nice and large and dark (as normally is on 400mg). Dozed for an hour in afternoon. Gave lesson to A-level pupil in late afternoon. Went to Library Theatre in evening, went to bed at 11 pm. (Woke up at 7:50 am).

Postscript (Day 67)

I have noticed few differences between how I am now that I am stabilised on 350mg and how I was on 400mg. The only possible differences I can think of are:

Slightly shorter sleeping at night,

Slight reduction in weight (currently 11st 9.5lbs),

Minutely better sexual function and

Possibly slightly more discontent.

Possibly slightly faster walking (brother thought so)

(All these are steps toward how I was before I got schizophrenia.)

More frequent involuntary movements (though still infrequent).

Reducing Medication II

About 11 years after the medication reduction mentioned in the previous section, I was on 300mg a day of amisulpride, 50mg in the morning and 250mg at night. However, I was getting dozier during the day and needed cans of the caffeinated drink *Monster* to feel reasonably awake and alert, and was sleeping despite the large amount of caffeine. So, I felt I could successfully achieve a medication reduction and now I switched to 25mg in the morning and 250mg at night, for a medication reduction of about 8%. The following is a diary of how I felt.

Day 1 Had 25mg less than normal in morning. Possibly slightly quicker movement in evening than usual, and thought of idea of using *Just A Minute* themes as themes for poetry (this idea never occurred to me before). However, could just be psychological. Very very early days.

Day 2 Woke about 5:10 am, breathing perhaps easier and warmer chest than expected. No caffeine so far, but sleepy despite medication reduction. Fine in Wetherspoons for lunch, though came over a bit hot after seeing N and agreeing to show her my drawing in 2 days time. E thought I was livelier and quicker moving on meeting me after work.

Day 3 Woke up at 6 am. Bit angry at E being unreasonable the night before. Maybe lifted legs over bed more easily. Slightly heightened hearing in library and vision in Marks and Spencer toilets, or so it seemed. Had a rest in afternoon as tired. Getting up from settee more easily?

Day 4 Woke up about 3:30 am having had difficulty going to sleep. Mind active but body tired. After waking, mind was very active, thinking a lot. Got up about 9 am. Made and received phone calls and visited N regarding picture for her. Tired in afternoon after reading T.H.E. Rang British Heart Foundation regarding collecting stuff in morning and put some things in bags for them. Went to bed at 9 pm.

Day 5 Woke up about 4:30 am after about 7 hours sleep. Listened to Desert Island Discs (Matt Smith). Mind less active than previous morning. Had lunch at Wetherspoons and chat with B2 in Library. Spoke with B3 in town. Did some sorting out in Dad's bedroom in morning. Shopping in afternoon. Felt reasonably okay. Went to bed 10:30 pm.

Day 6 Woke up about 5 am. Had briefly very slight sickness feeling (not sure if due to undercooked potatoes or medication reduction) but not sick. Brain quite lively after waking up. Slight ejaculation but not much. Visited Stockwood Discovery Centre. Bought honey, Luton Haiku book and hot drink and saw exhibition of excellent photographs. Updated poetry book to include N's comment and punctuation following B4's remarks. Read a lot of Daniel Tammet's book "Thinking In Numbers". Read more of this Luton Haiku book at a time than last one I read. Does this mean I have more mental stamina now that medication reduced? Got call that Mona Wall had died from her daughter.

Day 7 Woke around 6:50 am and got up around 7:50 am. Went shopping in late morning and met several people in town that I knew. The most interesting was N3, now in the Edwardian Care Home (168 Biscot Road?). She had reduced her medication recently and felt better because of it. Read some Haiku notes after lunch. Wrote 'Brother's Day' card for E for fun. Bit tired in afternoon. N3 expressed interest in my next poetry book (She had my third one).

Day 8 Woke up about 5:55 am. Thought of calling 5^(4^(3^(2^1))) the Thunderbirds Number! Rather tired though breathing seemed to be back to normal quiet shallow breathing. Watched TV programme "Holding Back The Years" in morning (unusually for me). Had big lunch in Hardware Café. They had The Daily Mail – an improvement – and did shopping, then later some sorting out. Tired in evening (extremely) but still filled and put out bins after reading two chapters of "Thinking In Numbers". Went to bed just before midnight.

Day 9 Woke up about 5:30 am. Breathing difficult. Before got up had an ejaculation. Did some sorting out and went for lunch and had medical check in small room in library. Need more exercise and to reduce cholesterol ratio. Chatted with B2 and read paper (The Guardian). Chatted also with F. Better able to think on feet and order at Bar in Wetherspoons than before I think (faster and more confident).

Day 10 Woke up at about 1:10 am due to being upset by E's unreasonable anger. Felt tired in day but saw GP and got some help concerning breathing (didn't take anything though). Finished "Thinking In Numbers" and did some preparing of bags for collection by British Heart Foundation. Stephen Hawking died, also Pi Day. Went to bed at 9 pm.

Day 11 Had a very good night's sleep – maybe best for many years in terms of being very deep. Watched TV, gave bags to British Heart Foundation man and had lunch and read about Stephen Hawking in The Sun. Read THE in the library and did shopping including fish in market (trout). Went for extra walk to Stockwood Discovery Centre and felt slimmer and livelier than for years. Read a bit in evening (Luton Haiku book). Went to bed at 11 pm.

Day 12 Woke up about 6:15 am after good sleep. Not all that lively but okay. Did some sorting out in morning and my books arrived – almost completely ready for selling as many as possible. Went to appointment with psychiatrist and got resistance from psychiatrist regarding medication reduction but he warmed a little to it in the end. Upset me rather though and took me hours to recover. Went to bed at about 11 pm.

Day 13 Woke up about 5:30 am. Got up about 8 am and went out to lunch at the Red Lion in the snow with E. Still feeling pretty sane and fine despite the psychiatrist's worries. Felt very good in fact – reminiscent of before I got ill. Read Luton Haiku a bit and had some Tortilla as a top-up to a small lunch. A customer swore this evening at the shop – a scary Saturday.

Day 14 Didn't sleep all that well and not sure when woke up. Had a dream/thoughts about GCHQ. Felt a bit better by end of Andrew Marr Show. Revised and republished and ordered 5 of my new book (tiny correction made). Read Sunday Times. Had a nice lunch including some cooking. Did some painting for N. Finished reading Haiku book (2012).

Day 15 Did some sorting of Mum's clothes, went out for lunch (Chicken Kiev) and met D and U. Found out about Pam Ayres coming to High Town Methodist Church. Did shopping and came home. Meal out with D2, E2 and E, went to Music Club. Was annoyed E didn't warn me of meal but got over it in an hour. Wrote poem to give to N at some point inscribed in book.

Day 16 Slept lightly but felt okay. Think D2 and E2 both have personality faults. Perhaps E2 best of bad lot. Sent video of her to N. Had lunch out, shopped, met Mariana briefly. Went to Discovery Centre, bought book. Went to town for meal with E and D2. Bored by them. Feeling fairly normal but more lively than for many years.

Days 17, 18, 19 Seemed more anxious and tried to manage by eating plenty. Almost got in a bit of a state of confusion on Wednesday before went out, but managed okay. Seemed more lively and slept only from about 11 pm to 5 am with 3:30 am wake up on night of Day 18/19. Seemed to follow Question Time and This Week better than for many years on evening of Day 19. According to E laughed more during it. Was anxious in morning about going to Wetherspoons and blood test but both went well apart from beggar standing in door of Wetherspoons asking for money (30p. I gave him 50p). Plus slightly scary seeing other bad types on way to Sainsbury's. Also slightly more active in consulting with E about dinner. N5 sent details of maths problem to me.

Day 20 Didn't sleep much. Worked on N5's maths problem (21 card trick which I generalised) during the day. Made good progress. Seem to have more drive even if anxious. Went for 3-mile walk.

Day 21 Again slept very little. During day worked on maths problem. Made good progress. Went to town and back for shopping. Worked quite well/semi-hard.

Days 22, 23 Main problem is very poor sleep, though managed to have a dream last night. Very tired in day. Anxiety perhaps lessening slightly. Finished all proofs in maths problem got from N5 (just over 6 pages long – N.B. last time did some meaty maths and wrote it up on computer like this was 2009 following slight medication reduction, and prior to that 2000 following coming off entirely. Latter 2 times sent it to others). Still pretty much no psychosis. Need to check mathematical literature to see if maths written up has been done before. Second biggest problem is? Tinnitus that has come on or is it hearing blood pumping in my right ear? Saw K's son U2 on Five Star Hotel on TV channel E4.

Day 24 Had slightly better sleep. Woke about 3:30 am after having had a dream (okay/nice this time). Think slept a bit more soundly than in previous few days.

Day 25 Had ECG, meal with B, errand for E, helped Uncle. Had slept badly following relatively demanding note from E. Some sorting out. Saw K's son U2 on TV.

Day 26 Slept slightly better – waking at 3:30 am and 6:30 am. Did some sorting in morning. Wrote Tanka. N5 says my maths somewhat beyond him so doesn't want to be co-author.

Day 27 (Birthday) Disruption from E and E2 and son moving furniture out of house, but went for meal with E later on (late lunch). Voices of neighbouring diners was loud, but E seemed more worked up about them. E thought I am now able to absorb and appreciate what others say more.

Day 28 Hadn't slept much at all last night. Went to Discovery centre for first Haiku book whilst cooking lunch. Prepared a bit for visiting University of Bedfordshire library, hopefully in a few days. Went to bed about 7:30 pm.

Day 29 Think had some sleep (reasonable amount?) after dull day yesterday. Had lunch out and visited Q, D3 and N6 in Tennyson Road in afternoon as was a little bored and lonely.

Winnie Mandela died. Slightly irritated* by K2 in Hardware Café saying "Good way to start the day" at lunchtime and remark about big meal. Perhaps he sleeps a lot till very late? Remembered playing snooker on own in 3rd year at University of Bath whilst watching it with Q – this never happened before now! Walked 3 times round Memorial Park. * - Wouldn't have been on old dose. He left loads on plate.

Day 30 Had gone to bed at 8:30 pm last night, slept a bit, including religious dream and woke up later and then another sleep and woke up later at about 5:10am so maybe best sleep for quite a few days. Possibly slightly depressed. Had an ejaculation. Got local beer from Discovery Centre, had lunch out – met T – annoyed me a little, not realising could not be a maths teacher. Met S from library. He is going to Leagrave library whilst library recovers from flood. Did shopping, read newspapers and two articles in Mathematics Today. Arranged for collection of bags by British Heart Foundation. Skimmed through 2 papers relevant to 21 card trick problem and wrote up a bit (adding to my article on the subject). Went to bed about 11 pm (Did painting in early evening).

Day 31 Woke up about 4 am after having reasonable sleep.

Day 32 Went to University of Bedfordshire library and downloaded 5 of 8 articles wanted. Did some more on painting for N. Chatted with B, especially about preparing for H's visit. Got me a bit anxious and didn't sleep much afterwards, but made some notes on ideas for how to cope.

Day 33 Took it fairly easy in morning. Went to Wetherspoons for lunch (sat with J). Found J nice as usual, but also rather nosey and intrusive. Maybe what he said caused more of a reaction/response in my brain than usual (pre medication reduction). Did shopping, saw Lego statues in Mall. Arranged to give radios+ to C2 and did more painting for N. Went to bed about 11:00 to 11:30 pm.

Day 34 Woke up about 6:23 am, so had best sleep for a while. Apparently, C2 doesn't sleep well and gets up at 5 am or even 4 am. Got up usual time (8:20 am alarm) and listened to some of Saturday Live. Felt have more restlessness/restless energy than on previous dose. Need to direct it well. Interestingly, eating satsumas seemed disgusting today – spat out flesh – just like when I was young or a child (taste buds going back to pre-illness ways?)

Day 35 Had ejaculation before semi-sleep – don't think slept properly, and ejaculation in morning too – first time two ejaculations in one night since been on meds. Was I a little excited by yesterday's events – lego, remark by person looking at them or maths reading (understood fairly well and possible thought of generalising if want) and so didn't sleep. Read 2 mathematical papers on card tricks, one completely thoroughly in morning. Think have more drive than on old dose. Read another paper in afternoon. Treated self to fizzy drink and chocolate as a reward. Did washing. Went to bed 10:30 pm.

Day 36 Slept very shallowly, if at all, but not really fully conscious till about 5:23 am. Got up about 8 am. Listened to Start The Week. Was a bit sharp/tetchy without meaning to be in Hardware Café – after I had asked for hot water he offered me a tea instead as he'd made a mistake and I said "no no" instead of "no thank you". Some youths and children blocked the path down to subway temporarily by chance and I got a whiff of cannabis - hope not affected. Did shopping, had a nice chat with woman member of staff at checkout –very nice, and had nice chat with partially sighted woman on seats in Arndale. Must go to Dunstable Library for Inter-Library Loans (no longer do for journals in Luton Central Library). Have more of a restless energy/hunger for activity. Went to bed about 11 pm after camomile tea (1).

Day 37 Woke up about 4:37 am after a dream. Had had proper sleep.

Day 38 - 41 Tried to manage to sleep by having one or two camomile teas (teabags) at night. N7's camomile not so good. Twining's camomile better. Seem to get about 4 or 5 hours a night with such a drink on average. Had quite a good time on 14th in London at B's 50th celebration. One mis? – hearing from waiter (maybe his accent).

Day 42 Had about 5 and a quarter hours sleep, waking up at 4:44 am with help of two Twinings teabags (camomile). Functioning reasonably well. Could have camomile tea in morning or even throughout day when H comes. Tinnitus doesn't seem to be there today. Went to bed about 11:15 pm. Was more able to engage with H on the phone I thought in a good way.

Day 43 Woke up about 5:56 am after having had two camomile tea (Twinings) bags so quite a good sleep. Maybe 6 hours or more. Did some sorting of cupboard under attic. Unfortunately, E a bit unpleasant and D3's Mum taken severely ill. Was quite articulate in my dispute with E – I was not so zombified that I couldn't argue.

Day 44 Did lots of sorting in morning. Went to Wetherspoons for lunch, got shopping and card for D3 and met N and walked with her for a bit. Tinnitus there again.

Day 45 Had not slept last night/only semi-conscious perhaps. Had good day in sunshine and emptying cupboard and filling it with journals. W (met him in town briefly) said he was unwell. K3 and N8 getting to know each other (K3 visiting

N8). A very active day. Felt cheerful and relaxed quite a bit. A very good day.

Day 46 Did not sleep last night, for third night in a row. Things making sleep difficult: pressure from E to sort things (he admits he does nothing), imminent visit by H, Dad's death (and loneliness in day)? Might be possible to cope in more favourable circumstances. Camomile not always effective in enabling sleep. Could a) increase dose to 25mg in the morning and 275mg at night or maybe b) 25mg in the morning and 262.5mg at night or c) take some sleeping tablet like zopiclone. Found out d) passionflower may help, also e) Valerian but N7 advises against Valerian and says passionflower taking requires approval of Doctor. If go for upping dose to 300mg total, could try going for 287.5mg total in more favourable circumstances. Tinnitus/Ear pulsing still there. Reading up on hypnotic drugs (e.g., zopiclone for sleeping problems) suggests sleep duration extended for only 15 mins and one adapts to the dose and not a long-term successful solution. N.B. started noticing effects as early as 2 days after initial medication reduction so may have effects very soon if put up to 25mg & 275mg. N.B. if put up to 25mg & 262.5mg for a total of 287.5mg then therapeutic threshold might lie between 300mg and 287.5mg, so not be crossed and may not sleep much better. Safest bet is 25mg & 275mg? Got plenty of sorting out done today (11 bags – most ever by quite a bit). Brain lively, able to talk well, think well and other benefits but can't sleep. E said on 14.4.18 my brain went from Sinclair to a Cray by reducing dose (at B's 50th Birthday Meal). Might it be possible to survive months of not sleeping and eventually would the brain return to a more normal sleeping pattern? How long would it take – 6 months/1 year? – took many months to recover from anti-psychotic given to me in '93 in Cheltenham and move to Loughborough/supervisors etc. Perhaps a reduction to 287.5mg would be easier to survive getting used to long term. Perhaps reduction by one-twelfth was too great.

(22.5.20 – above note is like Beethoven's Heiligenstadt Testament!)

Day 47 More relaxed than thought I would be, meeting H. Maybe better able to take in his rapid speech. But woke up at 1 am and decided to up dose by 12.5mg. Was calmer in night (that) afterwards. Had lunch with H, then met B2 for a chat.

Day 48 Had slept much better – till 4:30 am + a few more sleeps (brief) thereafter. Coped with H by escaping/resting.

Day 49 Scarcely slept at night, though at least one dream. Stressed after lunch with H and rested and read and went shopping. Telegraph (Sunday) has no TV schedule, but Maths At Cambridge news item! Slight struggle speaking – brain less active than on lower dose, but possibly better than on higher dose.

Day 50 Had slept quite well – till 5:26 am and then fairly dozy afterwards. Brain not too bad, but less lively than on lower dose. Read a bit of a Luton Haiku book in morning.

Day 51- 55 Slept very little each night, though perhaps better last night despite the cold coming in last day or so. Had a mild nightmare so slept a bit and may even have had a few hours of sleep. Is slightly higher dose building up in system? Today read a paper on 21-card-trick problem and updated my article. Didn't go out due to my cold. H left for a bit yesterday morning so a bit more peaceful for a while now.

Day 56 – 58 Didn't sleep much and cold progressed, except last night where was wheezing badly and slept/dozed right through till 8 am! Saw GP and they thought/said no infection or anything, just a continuation of the cold, though sounded really bad last night with very loud wheezing. Went shopping, had lunch out – walked down, bus back.

Day 59 Packed for hols but might not go. Slept till 4:xx am last night, not bad considering irritating behaviour by E (not willing to be in same room for more than a few moments once knew I still had cold) and holiday journey today (possible). Still slight tinnitus/ blood pumping near ear sound. Is slightly higher dose bedding in? New 50mg tablets are easier to divide up (already a groove down middle).

Postscript

I did go on holiday after all, though I was not well physically. I soon settled down to sleeping quite well on 287.5mg a day, 25mg in the morning and 262.5mg at night. Though somewhat more sleepy than on 275mg, I had a little more drive and liveliness than on 300mg and have had my two best years in terms of serious mathematical reading of textbooks and mathematical research since going on medication. Indeed, I have functioned at my best generally since going on medication, far exceeding any of the previous medicated years, and in my 'career' as a mathematician it is not exaggerating to say in the time since being on 287.5mg I have re-awakened as a mathematician from a state of torpor, and the reduction to 287.5mg instead of 300mg has been a great success.

Reducing Medication III

During the coronavirus pandemic I may have got the virus and several months after I was over the initial phase I was feeling very sleepy and resorting to cans of Monster again, so in mild desperation I decided to reduce the medication again, from 287.5mg to 281.25mg. The following diary tells the tale of this medication reduction.

Day 1 (17/8/20) Woke up 7:30am, felt physically better and less tired, but may be psychological. Bit tired. Went to bed 8:25pm.

Day 2 Woke up at 10:30pm, 1am and 6am, but slept okay apart from that. Did not feel much different from normal, except maybe more well and energetic. Had a green tea and a coke. Had idea to generalise zumkeller numbers to pattern in $\{-1,0,1\}^n$, Went to bed 11:15pm.

Day 3 Woke up at 6:50am. Feel more comfortable in the body, more energetic and younger. Had green tea, 2 Typhoo teas and a Monster due to sleepiness (relative) mentally. Did maths. Went to bed 11:10pm.

Day 4 Didn't sleep well (but did sleep (dreams once or twice) due to caffeine (too much)). Active morning, coding and rather overly hungry briefly in early afternoon. E visited and we had a late curry meal delivered. Went to bed around 11:15pm. No caffeine today.

Day 5 Woke up about 5:12am and thought a bit (had maths idea), got up about 7:40am. Missed breakfast due to extremely late meal night before, had no carbs at lunch and virtually no meal in evening due to E's zoom meeting. Went to bed about 11pm.

Day 6 Woke up 4:30am with headache - quite bad but got back to sleep and woke again at 9:40am. Had three teas (Typhoo) due to lack of mental awakeness! Chatted with B in Garden. Backed up hard disk. Went to bed at midnight.

Day 7 Had had a little difficulty getting to sleep, but woke up 7:04am. Did usual stuff plus backing up laptop. Went to bed 8:15pm. Woke 10:15pm. Then slept again some of time till 3:30am, then some sleep between then and 8am.

Day 8 Had a fairly enjoyable day eating out in covid times in Debenhams, bumping into D2 and walking with him round Stockwood Park (the short Uncle C-like route). Went to bed about 11pm.

Day 9 Woke up about 7:29am. Felt fairly okay. Researched 'convex' numbers (defined last night), and concave numbers, investigated Warwick Uni people in graphs and number theory. Had more elementary number theory ideas (including wiggly numbers) and Monster drink to celebrate Storm G. Went to bed at 11:45pm.

Day 10 Had difficulty sleeping due to Monster and worry from Storm G. Woke up at 6:30am and got up 7:45am. Felt somewhat tired from lack of sleep but did maths (wiggly numbers) and programming. Went to bed about 11pm.

Day 11 Woke up twice in night and went to toilet. Slept in the end till 9:50am! Had two cups of caffeinated tea and went to bed after watching Brideshead Revisited at 11:55pm.

Day 12 Woke up 4:10am. Then not sure slept and got up 7:40am. Did I have too much tea yesterday? Certainly, my conversation with E on zoom yesterday was more lively than for a long while. Had a small caffeinated drink – hope not too much caffeine. Shopped a bit, including trousers.

Day 13 Had poetry meeting online, some chat with E and face to face with B in evening. Had 1 cup of tea at 1:30pm, no other caffeine. Went to bed about 11pm?

Day 14 Woke up and went to the toilet at 2am and then slept till 6:30am. Slept a bit more (at least 1 dream per interval of time) and got up about 7:50am. Had a cup of tea about 10am and had a fairly lively (on my part) conversation with H on the phone – increased liveliness of mind due to medication reduction? Went to bed about 10:45pm.

Day 15 Woke up at 4:33am and had only light sleep thereafter. Dreamt of Mum and Dad in two separate dreams - Mum was in the kitchen, Dad at top of cellar steps. Programmed and watched Evan Carmichael on YouTube in morning. Thought of 2-valued numbers.

Day 16 Woke up at 4am. Had no caffeine. Went to bed at 9:30pm.

Day 17 Woke up 12:30am. Went to sleep once or twice more though suffering quite a bit of pain in ribs due to accident on sofa. Woke up 6:43am. Quite a good night's sleep 😊 Had a tea and coca cola before midday in town. Saw four people I know. Did some programming of V-shaped numbers. Watched zoo programme in evening. Went to bed 9:20pm.

Day 18 Woke up once or twice in night, but mostly slept until about 7am, then went back to bed due to tiredness and thought/slept till 9:43am! Had tea and coca cola in day. More testing of a conjecture. Went to bed at about midnight.

Day 19 Not sure slept much, though too sleepy/asleep/dozy to look at watch until after 6am. Got up about 7:30am. Got hair cut in Ashton Road 'Hope Barbers'. Was tired a lot of the day. Went to bed at 8:20pm.

Day 20 Woke up at 2:30am but slept (mostly) again till 6:55am. So had a lot of sleep. Had 2 cups of tea in early morning, phone call with H, walk in park and zoom call with E. Started writing LaTeX document on Ratio Graphs. Went to bed 11:10pm.

Day 21 Woke up about 6am. Not the best of sleeps but not bad either. Had a tea and green tea and had some good ideas for a proof. Had nice lunch, walk in afternoon – saw Q in Memorial Park. He is much the same as ever. Bit bored and went to bed at 8:15pm.

Day 22 Woke up at 1:27am and went to toilet and slept some more till about 7am. Got up 7:35am. Had 2 cups of Typhoo tea and with lunch in Red Lion and at home afterwards 2 Diet Cokes! Did maths research after emailing university people. Went to bed at 9:25pm.

Day 23 Amazingly, slept fairly well despite all that caffeine yesterday. Woke up once or twice in night without needing to go to toilet. Pain from hurting ribs about 11 days ago might be lessening (though still quite bad as lay down last night). Had a tea (and a V drink after took books to BHF). Did some of a proof and zoom calls with Mind and E. Went to bed about 10pm.

Day 24 woke about 4:xy am. Irritated by N2's message yesterday which I haven't read yet. It seems all she wants to do is sell me Fab and cake I don't want with almost no other conversation. Gave to charity shop and had 2 Typhoo teas and a green tea. Made good progress on mathematical proof of V-shaped numbers. Chatted to B over phone. Went to bed about 10pm.

Day 25 Woke up about 6:10am. Bit tired and dozed/slept/thought about proof till about 9:10am. Had a tea, green tea and Kombucha drink and washed-up and shopped and chatted with B2 in chance meeting in Tavistock Street. Zoomed with E and felt tired so went to bed at 8:10pm. E said I did a diatribe and it was a good thing and wouldn't have happened before reducing meds.

Day 26 Woke up at 4:57am, went to toilet and got up 7:40am after some light dozing/thought. Angry at E for discouraging me from doing maths and 'getting too excited' in the evening so that I can't sleep. Very annoyed. Met N2 in Memorial Park and gave her £10 for cake and 2 Fabs, plus new version of my first poetry book with her society. Had a Fab drink and tea in day. Finished important case in proof and did some testing of conjecture after bit of programming. Went to bed 11:10pm.

Day 27 Woke at 6:09am and got up at 8am. Spoke with E on phone in morning (he rang!) and on zoom in evening. Tested conjecture up to 10^8. Went to bed at 9:50pm.

Day 28 Woke up at 5:xy am and slept/dozed till 8:10am. Got paper, watched Andrew Marr, talked with H over phone, read paper, showered. Lunched at Moat house with B. Had a cup of tea in morning. Facebook chatted with N. Tired and went to bed 8:45pm.

Day 29: Woke at 4:xy am and slept/dozed till alarm at 7:32am. Got up at 8am. Had a tea and wrote a prose poem, took photos for E, bumped into S (formerly of XBX group) in town and chatted a bit. Breathing difficult in evening and went to bed early at 9:05pm.

Day 30 Woke at 3:57am and went to toilet. Slept/dozed till about 7:50am. Had green and ordinary tea. Got letter from M saying D had died. Zoomed at lunchtime, several photos for E. Bumped into G in town, zoomed with E in evening after reading some prose poems. Went to bed at 9:40pm.

Day 31 Woke at ?2:30am, went to the toilet and slept and dozed further till 8:10am. Took photos for E, sent card to M, bumped into B3 by Red Lion. Read more prose poems. Found out Darwin did 3 45minute walks a day. Went to bed at 10:15pm.

Day 32 Woke up early, went to D's funeral. Dropped off in town by vicar and his wife. Zoom meal with E (delivered curry). Read some prose poems. Went to bed 10:30pm. Had had two teas and a 'V' drink.

Day 33 Slept quite well till 4am but not thereafter. Seemed mentally more active and more awake than before reduction – maybe with bit more grit! Got up 7:20am. Read more prose poetry. Went to town in afternoon for sunshine. H2 is refusing to believe there is a virus (coronavirus). Continued testing conjecture, had two cups of tea. Went to bed at 9:20pm.

Day 34 Woke up at 3:38am and slept/dozed till 7:32am alarm. Got up at 7:40am. Listened to Saturday Live, Any Questions, went shopping, met B3 by chance in town, zoomed with E and met B face to face (with E on zoom). Had 2 teas and a Kombucha. Went to bed about ? 11:40pm.

Day 35 Woke up just before alarm (which is at 7:32am). Got paper, had two teas, watched Andrew Marr, spoke with H, read paper, met B3 in town as arranged and chatted for 3.5 hours. With help of Dean Grazioni and Evan Carmichael came up with my own rocking chair test. Went to bed 8:55pm.

Day 36 Woke at 12:50am and went to toilet. Thereafter slept till 6am and further sleep including dreams between 6am and 7am. Got up at 8:36am. Met C and B2 for lunch in Manor Park. Had tea and N2's bread and honey from B2 and went home and answered C's GCSE maths problem. Brief chat with E on zoom. Bit tired and went to bed at 9:55pm. Ejaculated for first time in months (rib problem and breathing problem getting better and meds reduction may have helped).

Day 37 Woke at 6:23am and got up at 8am. Felt quite good. Did photos for E, bit of LaTeX, zoom with Mind. Did brief trip to town (O now in care home) and did zoom with E. Went to bed at 9:50pm.

Day 38 Slept reasonably well and did a bit of LaTeX writing up of proof. Had haircut (short) in case of long lockdown. Had two teas and a Pepsi. B rang and we had a nice chat. C2 rang and irritated me by trying to dump a task on me. Bit angry. Went to bed about 10:15pm.

Day 39 Didn't sleep well due to a combination of Pepsi and C2 annoying me I think. Got up at 7:30am. Had two teas and did some sorting out in Breakfast room after a bit of LaTeX. Took stuff to BHF shop and zoomed with E and Luton Astronomical Society. Went to bed 11pm.

Day 40 Did not sleep well. Woke up and looked at watch at 1:xy am and 7:05am. At least dozed otherwise. Got up 7:20am. Maybe reacting to unsettling news of E's finances/still annoyed by C2. Did sorting out for at least 2 hours in Breakfast room, had green tea. 'Diagnosed' leak problem and addressed it. Went to town and back and chatted briefly with E. Felt lacklustre and tired (had been having low carb meals last 2 days) and perhaps also due to lack of sleep last 2 nights. Found out D3 has gone missing. Went to bed 8:15pm.

Day 41 Did not sleep particularly well. Woke up and got up at 4:57am, and don't think slept much till 7:32am alarm and getting up at 7:50am. Had carbs with both lunch and dinner and felt better because of it (had no carbs with some meals for last 2 days). Had green tea. Did zoom with poetry society and

E. Walked about 3 miles in park and to shop. Wrote start of "What's Next?" prose story. Went to bed 9:50pm.

Day 42 Slept better, woke up at 5:01am, slept/dozed with some dreams till 7:20am. Got up then. Did usual getting of paper, Andrew Marr, phone call with H, reading of paper. Didn't achieve much this day due to worrying about H. Went to bed about 9:15pm. Got up at 11:30pm and read email which put my worries to rest.

Day 43 Woke up several hours later and got up about 7:42am. Did usual routine including Evan Carmichael and rang B for brief chat, lunched in Red Lion, bumped into N3 and had brief chat. Rang E briefly, wrote some of a short story, "What's Next?" and watched Freddie Flintoff documentary. Went to bed 10:30pm.

Day 44 Woke up about 6am and slept/dozed till 8:40am when got up. Zoomed twice in day (Mind and E), brief chat with B, brief local shop. Had computer trouble and big anthology arrived in case of long lockdown. Had green tea. Went to bed 9:40pm.

Day 45 Woke up 6:42am and got up 7:30am. Had a green tea, went to library in new covid setup and had DietPepsi and did some good graph theory (fractious parties theorem) and wrote more of "What's Next?". Had a good time staying up till 11:15pm.

Day 46 Think Pepsi kept me awake till 1:xy am, then think slept till 6:wz am and got up about 7:50am. Did 2 mile walk and had green tea and Pepsi and ginseng tea. Restarted poetry with C, zoomed with E – he is experiencing a lot of stress/anxiety. Saw Question Time! Went to bed 12:10am.

Day 47 Woke at 7:13am. Wrote bit of short story, went to local shop, had green tea and Typhoo tea. Went to bed 12:45am!

Day 48 Woke up at 7:01am and dozed/rested till 8:50am and got up then. Had green tea, ginseng tea, Typhoo tea, saw E on zoom and B face to face. Went to bed 12:50am!

Day 49 Woke up about 8:40am. Had green tea, PG tips tea, watched Marr and Virtual London Marathon. Walked 3 miles in park including ¼ mile run. Went to bed 9:40pm.

Day 50 Slept better and did not wake until about 6:30am, and then further sleeping till 8:15am. Had 1 green tea and 1 Kombucha in town. Wrote a bit of the short story.

Day 51 Hardly slept at all but think did dream a little. Think due to difficult breathing and/or Kombucha. Got up 8:45am. Had green tea, 2 zooms and phone call from E2. Went to bed 9:45pm.

Day 52 Slept till about 3:30am, then dozing/sleeping till 8:15am. Might have done better after 3:30am, but bit worried about Facebook post. Had green tea and PG tips tea and walk to town where saw H2, and pigeons getting fed in St. George's Square and on way home saw N4 of Tennyson Road. Wrote more of a short story. Went to bed 11:30pm.

Day 53 Not sure slept much – opened eyes and looked at watch at 6:10am and got up 7:50am. Need to reduce caffeine I think. Had just 1 green tea and no other caffeine. Wrote 2 poems and talked with B, zoomed with E, walked to town and back. Went to bed 12:20am.

Day 54 Had left heating on by accident – woke up at 4:xy am and then slept to exactly 7:32am – pressed watch button a fraction of a second after 7:32:00am when alarm due to go off, hence scarcely a sound – quite a coincidence. Had 1 green tea, went for a 2-mile walk. Went to bed 11:45pm.

Day 55 Woke up about 7am. Further rest/dozing till 9am. Had 1 green tea, walked 2.5 miles, briefly chatted with Q and his aunt and D2. Zoomed with E, chatted with B. Went to bed 10:50pm.

Day 56 Woke up at 5:xy am and mostly awake but some sleep from then till 8:35am. Tired. Talked with H, did 1 mile walk and had 1 green tea, did other usual Sunday things. Went to bed 10pm.

Day 57 Woke up 2:xy am and dozed till 7am, then thought till 7:32am alarm, got up 7:50am. Had 1 green tea and went to town and back. Chatted to a N5 (former librarian) from Mind. Found out from him that the really mentally ill guy I know is N6. Went to bed 9:45pm.

Day 58 Woke up 5:09am and slept/dozed/thought till 7:32am. Had Kombucha (1), zoomed with Mind and E, chatted with B. Went to bed 10:40pm.

Day 59 Woke at 6:xy am and rested/dozed till 8:54am. Had 1 green tea, went to town and back, read some poetry. Went to bed 9:45pm.

Day 60 Woke at midnight and again at 4:xy am. Not sure slept much after that. Got up 8:30am. Had 1 green tea, went to library and got Birthday card, chatted with B, zoomed with E, got reply from academic willing to collaborate. Went to bed 11:20pm.

Day 61 Woke up 2:xy am and again at 4:xy am, but did not get much sleep, thinking about maths and the academic. Got up 6am to empty oven dish, then back to bed. Then up properly about 7:40am. Had 1 green tea, stayed in for plumber and didn't walk. E came back in evening. Went to bed 12:05am.

Day 62 Woke up 6:12am and rested/dozed till 7:50am. Had 1 green tea and lots of company from E. Went to bed 10pm.

Day 63 Woke up at 2am and had 1 dream at least between then and 7:12am, but not much sleep. Got up 7:28am. Had no caffeine, plenty of time with E, chatted with B in park etc. Walked to town and back. Went to bed 10pm.

Day 64 Woke up at about 3:30am and again at about 5:30am. Dozed/slept/rested till 7:32am alarm. Had a very sleepy day, walked to Sainsbury's and back and got and drank Diet Coke. Tidied up breakfast room table, did a bit of LaTeX. Saw E and H at virtual Music Club. Went to bed at 11:40pm.

Day 65 Woke up once and slept through alarm at 7:32am and got up at 8:55am. Had 1 green tea and zoom with Mind and E and chatted with B. Went to bed 11:30pm.

Day 66 Did not sleep (partly anxiety about zoom with academic). Got up 7:58am. Might have to increase dose to 283.33mg? Interacted with Academic, zoomed with E too and chatted with B. Went to bed about 10:45pm.

Day 67 Did not sleep well – stressed and excited by interaction with academic. Went to toilet at 5:xy am and got up at 7:10am. Walked to town and back, zoomed with E – he said haiku I wrote today was 10 out of 10, my best ever poem, and had thoughts on platform numbers. Spoke to S in town – he 'has had enough' (what with one friend in care home, the other beaten up and in hospital) . Went to bed 11pm.

Day 68 Did some programming, LaTeX and maths and went to town and back. Chatted with B, had 1 green tea. Went to bed 12pm. **Started on 283.33mg today.**

Day 69 Woke up 4:xy am and got up 7:50am, didn't hear alarm and had a dream, but don't think slept much. Was tired in afternoon but felt better after sweet drink and did some LaTeX and maths. Had no caffeine. E not well so only chatted for a moment on phone. Went to corner shop. Went to bed 10:40pm.

Day 70 Slept well till woke up at 5:20am, rested/dozed till 7:30am. Walked to town after feeling tired after lunch, got a Diet Pepsi, wrote haiku, zoomed with E, chatted with B and H and did some LaTeX. Had drive and irritation with B (unspoken) in evening. Went to bed 10:55pm.

Day 71 Woke up at 6:17am and got up about 8am. Felt good. Had 1 green tea, went shopping, had Kombucha, E made a surprise visit and zoomed with Music Club and saw Richard Stilgoe. Facebooked with N. Went to bed 11pm.

Day 72 Woke up about 5:xy am and then did some sleeping through 7:32am alarm and woke up 8:05am. Lots of chatting with E – mostly E talking, walked 3 miles, said Hello to T, did a bit of LaTeX. Had a green tea. Went to bed 11pm.

Day 73 Dozed? Till 5am and then slept till about 8:30am. Think caffeine yesterday delayed sleep. Had a green tea, chats with E, zoom with academic. Thought about sequence academic invented.

Day 74 Didn't sleep well till about 2am when got up to go to toilet. Slept then till 7:10am. Felt very tired and didn't do much, but spoke with C2 on the phone, E on zoom, B on phone. Went to bed 11pm.

Day 75 Woke up 4:xy am and again at 6:55am. A better sleep - due to no caffeine? Had quiet day, worked on Optimizing

Schizophrenia book and bit of maths. Went to bed about 11:40pm.

Day 76 Woke at 3:51am and 7:53am. Quite a good sleep. Had a green tea in morning. Rather tired from late morning shopping with E. Zoomed with poetry society and more shopping with E + walk with B to what was Stockwood High School. Went to bed about midnight.

Day 77 Woke up about 5:30am and got up 7:10am. Walked for 2 miles in park. Talked to H on phone. Spoke to K in street. No caffeine. Went to bed 10:30pm.

Day 78 Woke up 4am and again about 7am, dreamt a bit till 8:25am. Chatted with E (he was around most of day), also with E2 on phone and B on phone, got stuff installed on newish laptop. Attended Music club zoom too. Went to bed 11:50pm.

Day 79 Woke up at 6am and slept some more between then and 9:19am, when woke up properly. Had a Diet Pepsi and hot chocolate in Debenhams due to imminent lockdown. Zoomed with E. Spoke to T. Went to bed at midnight.

Day 80 Did not sleep till after 1am with maths ideas. Woke up at 6am after cry next door – Biden win? and had ejaculation. Got up 7am. Had green tea in afternoon after lunch in Debenhams (pre-lockdown treat) and zoomed with academic & E. Phone calls with E2 and B and C2. C2 irritated me again. Went to bed at about 11:30pm.

Day 81 Woke up at 6:xy am and later slept through 7am alarm and got up 7:50am. No caffeine. Zoomed with E, walked in park and towards town about 2 miles. Did more maths. Went to bed 12:05am.

Day 82 Woke up about 6am, and then more rest and sleep till 10am! Had a green tea and wrote a poem about Trump, walked about 2 miles, Facebook chatted with N and did a bit of maths. Went to bed 11:50pm.

Day 83 Woke up about 7am. Walked 2.5 miles, saw Biden win, zoomed with E, did a little maths. Went to bed 10:30pm.

Day 84 Woke up about 7am. Thought about maths and got up about 8:30am. No caffeine but did some programming and math and zoomed with B and spoke with H. Walked 3 miles. Went to bed 11pm.

Day 85 Woke up at 6:16am and slept/dozed till past 9am. Had a Kombucha, chatted to B3 in town in chance meeting – police woman told us to start walking! Did more maths, spoke briefly to E. Went to bed 11:10pm.

Day 86 Woke up a little before 6am. Got up about 7:50am. Walked in park 2 miles and chatted to 2 older people about poetry – one seemed to know I was a poet. Zoomed with Mind and E. Did some maths and programming. Bit anxious about asserting self with academic. Went to bed about 11pm.

Day 87 Woke at 3:16am and rested/dozed till 7:30am. Anxious about academic. Had green tea, walked to Wilko and back, zoomed with academic (went well, relieved) and quick chat with E. Went to bed about 11pm.

Day 88 Woke just before 7am and got up 7:45am. Had ordinary tea and did some shopping in town and quite a bit of maths, plus brief call and zoom with E. Went to bed 12:10am.

Day 89 Woke up 7:30am. Walked a mile in park and to town and back, met by chance N2. M rang and B too. All irritated me a bit. Had 1 ordinary tea. Went to bed 11pm.

Day 90 Woke at 6:45am and had further dream (about Trump) before getting up at 8:55am. Zoomed with E and chatted whilst on a walk with B. Biden has reached 306 electoral college votes. Went to bed 10:38pm. No caffeine.

Day 91 Woke at 3:12am and 6:36am and finally woke at 8:05am and got up. Talked to H, got paper, read paper, saw Marr, walked 1.5 miles, did some maths and LaTeX. Went to bed 10:55pm.

Day 92 Worried about H and did not sleep till after 1:50am, when went to toilet. Woke up just before 7am. Sent and received email with H. Had an ordinary tea, walked 3 miles to Slip End and back. Didn't feel like doing much today. Think recovering from stress of worrying about H. Went to bed 9pm.

Day 93 Slept until 6:30am and then further dozing/sleep till 8:20am alarm when got up. Did some maths, shopping, zoom with E and Mind. A stressful day. Went to bed 8pm.

Day 94 Did not sleep at all due to interaction with Neighbours. Got up 8:08am. Rested a lot, did not zoom with Academic, chatted with B on phone, very briefly with E and did small amount of maths. Went to bed 10:38pm.

Day 95 Woke up at 12:xy am, 4:wz am and 6:18am and finally up at 8:25am. Slept well with a dream about a conference! Chatted with N2, B2 and Mr T2 on walk to Manor Park and back (2 miles). Went to bed 12:10am.

Day 96 Did not sleep till after 1:40am. Slept through alarm till 9:30am. Walked 1.5 miles, had an ordinary tea, read Built To Serve by Evan Carmichael, spoke with E2. Spoke briefly with E. Went to bed roughly 11:50pm.

Day 97 Woke up at 6:48am. Had further dream between then and 8:20am when got up. Had an ordinary tea.

Day 98 Got up at 8:38am and had an ordinary tea and got paper, chatted to H, saw Marr, read paper. Went for a 1.5-mile walk. Did some programming and maths. Went to bed 12:45am.

Day 99 Got up at 7:47am. Had an ordinary tea. Did some maths and a 3-mile walk. E2 and B rang. Went to bed about 11:30pm.

Day 100 Woke up about 9:50am. Did a 2.5-mile walk, had an ordinary tea, zoomed with E for 3 hours, did some LaTeX and programming. Went to bed 11:15pm.

Postscript

I ended the diary after 100 days as I seemed fairly stable on 283.33mg and sleeping better than on 281.25mg. Since being on a dose of 283.33mg I have functioned at my best yet on medication, collaborating with an academic and producing more than 60 pages of mathematical typed-up output and conducting further reading of mathematical text books and continuing to work mathematically and stay reasonably sane despite having problems with the academic that upset me a great deal. I hope to publish some mathematical papers arising from work done on this dose in the fairly near future.

Religion

St. Dymphna is the patron saint of those who suffer from mental illnesses. See, e.g., Wikipedia on the World Wide Web.

From notes provided by a psychoeducation group at Calnwood Court, Luton:

Many mystical or religious experiences contain elements that in another context would be deemed psychotic – e.g., St Paul was converted to Christianity after falling off his horse in a flood of light and hearing a voice questioning him (Acts 9:1-8).

Research

From the SAGB leaflet 'The Mental Diseases that Attack Mankind', October 1996:

There are almost 80,000 sufferers from schizophrenia in hospital in Britain now.

From the SAGB leaflet 'A Plea to all General Practitioners to treat Schizophrenic patients as medically ill', received in the year 2000:

Very often the patient has to stay on neuroleptics for life or risk a worsening of his illness. He may suffer severe side effects from the medication such as movement disorders and live an unsatisfactory, often zombie-like existence, in poor and unsuitable accommodation and with no job.

Outcome in schizophrenia is not significantly better now than it was early in the century.

From The Association of the British Pharmaceutical Industry's booklet 'Target Schizophrenia', 1997:

One of the tragedies of schizophrenia is that the common forms afflict people in their prime years, usually between the ages of 15 and 45. Men and women are affected equally, but the age of onset tends to be slightly earlier in men. Schizophrenia associated with major delusions is about ten times less common, has a later onset (40-55 years) and affects women slightly more often than men. (A graph shows the incidence of paranoid schizophrenia rising from a low level in the early thirties, peaking around age 45 and back down to low levels at age 55.)

From SAGB booklet 'Can you tell me something about Schizophrenia':

Schizophrenia is a more severe illness in males.

From SAGB booklet 'A Beginner's Booklet about Schizophrenia':

The illness can start at any age from childhood to old age.

From 'Schizophrenia and depression', a booklet produced by the National Schizophrenia Fellowship in January 1998:

Antipsychotic medication often causes sleepiness and may slow down the person's ability to think.

From The Observer Magazine, 21st May 2000, p. 45-46:

Professor Leff believes that 'if a person experiencing voices doesn't find them difficult to live with, and isn't impelled towards dangerous acts like suicide or homicide by them, who are we to say that they should be got rid of?'

From an article by Dr Raj Persaud, date unknown:

Schizophrenia is the most serious nonfatal illness.

From New Scientist, 3rd March 2001, page unknown, 'Soothing the Mind':

Researchers have suspected for a while that oestrogen helps protect against schizophrenia, because women suffer a milder version of the disease than men and it usually strikes them in later life. (The research in this article shows that oestrogen does help treat schizophrenia.)

From The Observer Magazine, 19th August 2001, p. 45-46:

The incidence of schizophrenia in the population as a whole is one in 100, but that figure shields a striking disparity. Fathers in their mid-twenties stand just a one-in-250 chance of having a schizophrenic child – compared to a one-in-46 risk for 50-year-old fathers.

From Psychiatric Bulletin (2002) 26: 295-298, 'Unemployment rates among patients with long-term mental health problems':

Unemployment among people with long-term mental health problems increased from 80% in 1990 to 92% in 1999, and the unemployment rates among those with a diagnosis of schizophrenia increased from 88% in 1990 to 96% in 1999, despite a decreasing rate of general unemployment for the majority of that period.

From SAGB Newsletter, Spring/Summer 2002, p. 1:

The outcome for schizophrenia has been said to be little better now than at the beginning of the twentieth century. Patients are expected to become only partially better.

From The Observer, OM Magazine, 'Distant Voices' by Oliver James:

Poor people are about twice as likely as the rich to suffer schizophrenia ... Schizophrenia is less common in developing nations and the illness tends to last longer and to be more severe in rich, industrialised nations compared with poor, developing ones. In fact, if you go mad in a developing nation you are 10 times less likely to have any recurrence of the illness – a huge difference, also nothing to do with genes.

From The Times Higher, October 3rd 2003, p. 29, 'Stalled on the brink of insight':

In any given year, 99.97 percent of those diagnosed with schizophrenia will not be convicted of serious violence.

From Mind in St. Albans leaflet:

The World Health Organisation has found depression to be the world's second highest cause of death.

Only 13 percent of people with significant mental health problems are in employment.

From Scientific American, January 2004, p. 38-45:

Of the roughly 1 percent of the world's population stricken with schizophrenia, most remain largely disabled throughout adulthood. ... Many undergo a decline in IQ when the illness sets in. ... Roughly 60 percent live in poverty. ... Antipsychotics stop all symptoms in only about 20 percent of patients. ....In the past few years, suspicion has fallen on deficiencies in the neurotransmitter glutamate.

Certain functions, such as the ability to form new memories either temporarily or permanently or to solve complex problems, may be particularly impaired.

Abstainers from substance abuse behave no more violently than the general population.

What physicians diagnose as schizophrenia today may prove to be a cluster of different illnesses, with similar and overlapping symptoms.

From The Observer, OM magazine, 30th May 2004, p. 57:

Unfortunately a quarter of patients are not helped by drugs at all and around 15 percent of all schizophrenics eventually commit suicide. Where the drugs do work, the reduction in symptoms is not large, only a 15 per cent to 25 per cent decrease.

From *New Scientist, 24th July 2004, p. 14, 'Creative spark can come from schizophrenia'*:

Why has schizophrenia not been eradicated from our genes? The answer might be because people with mild symptoms engage both sides of their brain and use more of it. This allows them to excel at creative endeavours. ... "I have no doubt that the genes for schizophrenia are associated with the genes for creativity," Shelley Carson at Harvard University says.

From The Guardian, date unknown, 'Met admits stigmatising mentally ill' by John Carvel:

A review by police and NHS chiefs in London said: "We recognise that people who experience mental illness are far more likely to be a victim of crime than a perpetrator."

From *The Guardian*, Tuesday October 25th 2005, p. 35, 'Opening a debate on schizophrenia':

"Clear evidence for brain-disabling and long-term damage caused by the use of psychotropic drugs was presented. What was particularly staggering to me was the wealth of research studies that show this, stretching back to the 1960s, which all the latest neurological test procedures are confirming." – Sue Johnson, Director, James Nayler Foundation.

"A person with schizophrenia is four times more likely than average to die from a respiratory infection. It is essential this and every autumn that GPs invite patients with severe mental health conditions to get immunised against flu." - Dr Alan Cohen, GP, Angela Greatley, Sainsbury Centre for Mental Health and six others.

From *New Scientist*, 19th November 2005, p. 52, Nancy Andreasen speaking:

"My own work has already shown that people with schizophrenia have an ongoing loss of brain tissue. The question is: why? Is it because of the disease itself? Is it because of the side effects, or even toxicity, from medication?"

From Schizophrenia Bulletin, Volume 32, Number 4, October 2006, Attitudes of Mental Health Professionals Towards People With Schizophrenia and Major Depression, by C. Nordt, W. Rossler and C. Lauber, 709-714:

"The reaction to the vignettes did not differ between professionals and the public. Both groups reacted with greatest social distance toward the person in the schizophrenia vignette, whereas between the depression and the non-case vignettes no difference was found."

- Here 'social distance' measures the willingness to interact with the person described in various social situations, e.g., whether you would like having your children marry someone like them.

From Perceptions Magazine, Spring 2007, p. 4:

In their book New Thinking about Mental Health and Employment (Radcliffe) the researchers Grove, Secker & Seebohm reported that the unemployment rate for people with schizophrenia is close to 95%.

From Schizophrenia Digest, Spring 2007, p. 19:

'Most people with schizophrenia improve over time: study':

They found that about 75% of patients actually improved over time based on this assessment method, and only a minority of patients appeared to deteriorate.

Source unknown:

In a study by Robert Rosenheck of 1438 patients with schizophrenia, nearly 15% were competitively employed and 13% worked in sheltered jobs. The rest were unemployed.

From *The Independent*, 11.09.08, 'My Son, The Schizophrenic':

An American doctor had described schizophrenia as being to mental illness what cancer is to physical ailments. The average age for the onset of schizophrenia is 18 in men and 25 in women.

From *The Observer*, 'Molecule Of Motivation Excels at Task':

Dopamine is less about pleasure and reward than about drive and motivation.

From *The Observer*, 12.04.09, 'Four psychiatric patients dying each day in NHS care':

1,282 people in England died in what it calls "patient safety incidents in mental health settings" in 2007-08. Another 913 patients suffered severe harm or permanent injuries in such incidents.

From *Building a Healthier Britain* (BBC Radio 4, 2005):

A couple of genes have been found to double the chance of getting schizophrenia if you have the wrong version of them. They are "neuregulin" on chromosome 8 and "Dysbindin" on chromosome 6.

From *The Guardian, 31/5/10 'Why teenagers can't concentrate: too much grey matter'*:

"We knew that the prefrontal cortex of young children functioned in this chaotic way but we didn't realise it continued until the late 20s or early 30s." This shows that my brain was probably still developing in my prodrome phase of schizophrenia or when I got schizophrenia at age 31, and so even at that late age it does not contradict the idea that it is a developmental disorder.

From *SZ Magazine Spring 2010:*

Omega-3 fish oils may prevent schizophrenia.

Mice with schizophrenia have been developed.

From *The Depression Report: A New Deal for Depression and Anxiety Disorders*:

"...schizophrenia, the most difficult of all mental illnesses, ..."

Percentage suffering from mental illness:	All	Women	Men
Psychosis (mainly schizophrenia)	0.5	0.6	0.5
Depressive episode	2.6	2.8	2.3
Generalised anxiety	4.4	4.6	4.3
Phobias	1.8	2.2	1.3
Obsessive compulsive disorder	1.1	1.3	0.9
Panic attacks	0.7	0.7	0.7
Other (mixed depression and anxiety)	8.8	10.8	6.8
Any of the above	16.4	19.4	13.5

Source: Psychiatric Morbidity Survey, 2000. Adults aged 16-75. More than one condition is possible.

From SZ Magazine, Winter 2009:

Schizophrenia is sometimes referred to as "youth's greatest disabler".

Trials are underway to test new drugs for schizophrenia that improve cognition.

From SZ Magazine, Winter 2010:

'Those with psychosis prone to heart disease':

Reason for this: As well as smoking and inactive lifestyle, it is likely due to the isolating, debilitating nature of mental illness.

'Schizophrenia risk rises with father's age: Study':

"...the odds of developing schizophrenia increased by 30% for each 10-year increase in paternal age."

From SZ Magazine, Fall 2009, p. 41, 'Schizophrenia drug could beat cancer':

"...antipsychotic medicines may also destroy cancer cells, explaining one of the mysteries of mental health: why schizophrenia patients have lower rates of cancer."

From Schizophrenia Digest, Summer 2008, p. 26:

About 50% of people diagnosed with schizophrenia do not understand they are ill.

From Schizophrenia Digest, Spring 2008, p. 16:

"... people with serious mental illnesses – including schizophrenia – die at least 25 years earlier than the general population, largely due to preventable medical conditions such as diabetes, cardiovascular disease, and respiratory and infectious diseases."

From All in the Mind, BBC Radio 4, 4th October 2011:

"patients with severe mental ill health die up to 20 years prematurely compared to an age-matched population"

This is supported by my personal experience. I know of five schizophrenics who used to attend Befrienders (now Luton Mind) who have died. Their ages at death were 27, 34, 47, 54 and 59.

From Schizophrenia Digest, Fall 2008, p. 13:

People with schizophrenia struggle to concentrate, remember and learn.

From Schizophrenia Digest, Fall 2008, page 36:

Memory, attention and problem solving are severely affected in about nine out of 10 persons with schizophrenia – making it difficult for many of them to have active lives.

From Schizophrenia Digest, Fall 2008, p. 44:

Americans see those with schizophrenia as 'damaged' in some essential way and, therefore, likely to be violent. However, when applied to depression, genetic arguments have very different connotations: they are associated with social acceptance.

From SZ Magazine, Summer 2009, p. 40:

'Cognition already seriously impaired in first episode of schizophrenia'

From SZ Magazine, Spring 2009, p. 35:

Between 40 and 50 percent of people with schizophrenia live with their families.

From Schizophrenia Digest, Winter 2008, p. 21:

'People with schizophrenia think logically':

The people with schizophrenia significantly outperformed the controls, leading the researchers to believe that on a straightforward interpretation, people with schizophrenia reason more logically than those without the illness, either because they are better at logic or because they are worse at common sense.

From *Conversations with Bill MacPhee – Ravi*, SZ magazine:

Half of the homeless in Toronto have schizophrenia.

From *Conversations with Bill MacPhee – Tammy*, SZ magazine:

She has to put in 5 hours work for every 2 hours a normal person puts in in her studies, as it is difficult for her to take in information.

From *Conversations with Bill MacPhee – Dr Peer*, SZ magazine:

What we have to get through to them is that this is something like diabetes, for example, in which they are going to have to be on something all their life and there's no way around that.

From http://news.bbc.co.uk/1/hi/health/6971037.stm , 2nd September 2007:

A drug which targets glutamate rather than dopamine in the brain has proved successful in treating schizophrenia. This may lead to the development of a third generation of drug treatments for schizophrenia.

From *All in the Mind*, BBC Radio 4, 29.06.10:

According to this programme Schizophrenics have difficulty or do not see the Necker Cube illusion (see https://en.wikipedia.org/wiki/Necker_cube). I have schizophrenia and was able to see it.

From *The Independent*, 'Living with Psychosis: I'm mad, but not bad', 13th July 2010:

My official one is "paranoid psychosis", but various psychiatrists have suggested I use "nervous disorder" or even the slightly odd "acute disability" when I raise it with potential employers. According to Mind, more than half of people would not employ the person they thought was the best candidate during an interview if they had disclosed a mental health problem.

From an advert in Schizophrenia Bulletin:

"In patients with bipolar mania, psychotic symptoms are prevalent in approximately 50% of manic episodes."

From SAGB Newsletter, Summer 1999, p. 27:

The suicide rate for psychotic patients has risen from about 2% in a Royal College publication of 1967 to the present figure 10-12% and is thus phenomenally high. This increase in suicides is due, I believe, to a combination of the drug treatment and the lack of the asylum of the old hospitals.

From Schizophrenia Bulletin, Volume 31, Number 2, April 2005:

p. 196:

"We conclude that high IQ does not protect against positive symptoms of psychosis nor against specific cognitive impairments, which are present in almost every case of first-episode psychosis."

p. 205:

Those with no family history of schizophrenia and paternal age > 33 years may form a distinct type of schizophrenia (Paternal age related schizophrenia or PARS). "PARS cases had superior WAIS-R IQ scores, greater medication free positive symptoms, and less deficit syndrome schizophrenia than familial cases."

p. 485:

'Rivastigmine improves memory of schizophrenia patients: a behavioural and ERP study'

From *Henry's Demons*, published in 2010:

p. 95: 60% of males with schizophrenia attempt suicide at least once.

p. 97: "In the US, HIV (including AIDS) research receives $2241 per person affected, compared to just $75 per person affected by schizophrenia."

"In the 1972 US Presidential Election, the revelation that Senator Thomas Eagleton had received electric shock treatment and had once checked himself into a hospital because of psychological problems was enough to get him sacked as the Democratic Vice-Presidential candidate."

p. 189: "A schizophrenic patient is a hundred times more likely to kill himself or herself than to kill somebody else." ... "About 8% of offenders who murder or attempt a murder have schizophrenia, and schizophrenic patients are four times more likely to be involved in violent incidents than people who have not been diagnosed as having a psychosis."

From Mensa Magazine, March 2018, p. 24:

Kynurenine is a molecule that is formed in the brain. Researchers at the University of Maryland School of Medicine report that people with schizophrenia have high levels of this compound in their brains compared to levels found in people unaffected by it. The researchers also found high levels of Kynurenine to be associated with less REM (or dream) sleep. They conclude that high levels of Kynurenine disrupt sleep and thus, could become a target for novel therapies for schizophrenia and in particular, the disrupted sleep pattern that is so often associated with this disorder.

Schizophrenia Caused by Illegal Drugs

From the leaflet *All about Schizophrenia* by South Essex Partnership NHS Foundation Trust: "Illegal drugs may trigger the illness in some people. For example, heavy cannabis users are six times more likely to develop schizophrenia than non-users."

Schizophrenia Journals

Those who really want to know a lot about schizophrenia and are prepared to work at it may be interested in the Journal *Schizophrenia Bulletin* at a price of £111 for 6 issues in the year 2020. This contains the interesting First Person Account/Personal Account which is very readable, cover art by schizophrenics as well as harder-to-read academic articles. See www.academic.oup.com/schizophreniabulletin .

Another source of information is http://www.psychiatryonline.org/ .

Service Users' Experiences

From *Challenging Discrimination Together*, Monday 12th July 2010, Hightown Community Sport and Arts Centre, Luton, Talk by Diana Jakubowska:

One service user said, "I prefer to say I've been in prison – it's easier to explain and they give me a chance".

From *Time to Change* campaign in the *Daily Mirror* Special Feature:

When Stuart Baker-Brown from Dorset was diagnosed with schizophrenia he was told he had to accept that it was unlikely he'd ever work again and he'd be viewed as a potential threat to society.

From Schizophrenia Digest, Summer 2008:

Doctors told him (Dean) he would probably end up living in a group home, and that a job and a relationship were unlikely.

Smoking

When I was in a mental hospital last I asked all the staff and inpatients whether they smoked. Out of 14 patients, only two didn't smoke whereas among 10 staff only two smoked.

Stress

How Stress Can Affect Your Body (From *Awake!* Magazine, no.1 2020, pages 6-7):

Nervous system

Your nervous system causes hormones such as adrenaline and cortisol to be released. These increase your heart rate, your blood pressure, and the glucose levels in your blood – all of which enable you to respond quickly to danger. Too much stress can lead to – irritability, anxiety, depression, headaches, insomnia.

Musculoskeletal system

Your muscles tense up to protect you from injury. Too much stress can lead to – body aches and pains, tension headaches, muscle spasms.

Cardiovascular system

Your heart beats faster and harder to distribute blood throughout your body. Blood vessels dilate or constrict to direct blood where your body needs it the most, such as in your muscles. Too much stress can lead to - high blood pressure, heart attack, stroke.

Respiratory system

You breathe faster to take in more oxygen. Too much stress can lead to – hyperventilation and shortness of breath, as well as panic attacks in those who are prone to them.

Endocrine system

Your glands produce the hormones adrenaline and cortisol, which help the body react to stress. Your liver increases your blood-sugar level to give you more energy. Too much stress can lead to – diabetes, lower immunity and increased illness, mood swings, weight gain.

Gastrointestinal system

The way your body processes food is disrupted. Too much stress can lead to - nausea, vomiting, diarrhoea, constipation.

Reproductive system

Stress can affect sexual desire and function. Too much stress can lead to – impotence, disrupted menstrual cycle.

Symbols to look out for when seeking an employer

Mindful Employer – see https://www.mindfulemployer.dpt.nhs.uk/ .

Positive About Disabled People.

A job that is possibly very suitable for someone who knows a lot about mental illness is Referrals Coordinator at a local Mind centre.

Symptoms

From http://www.bbc.co.uk/health/conditions/mental_health/disorders_schiz3.shtml, a site which is no longer available, accessed on 26/07/05:

Positive symptoms: abnormal experiences – such as delusions and hallucinations

Negative symptoms: loss of normal behaviour, including emotions, energy, interest, creativity and activity.

From http://www.chovil.com/graph3.html , a page which no longer exists:

Positive symptoms: Delusions, Hallucinations, Disorganised Speech, Catatonia.

Negative symptoms: Affective flattening, Alogia, Avolition, Anhedonia.

Cognitive symptoms: Attention, Memory, Executive functions (e.g., abstraction)

Mood symptoms: Dysphoria, Suicidality, Hopelessness.

The Author's Relevant Mathematical Ideas

<u>Diminished capacity to focus/concentrate with schizophrenia:</u>

Since getting schizophrenia the author thinks he has been less able to spend lots of time on any one thing. Thus, if the n distinct activities engaged in during waking hours in a day (or some other longer period) are engaged in for times $t_1, t_2, \ldots, t_n$ and $t = t_1 + t_2 + \ldots + t_n$ then the 'repeat rate' or 'incidence of coincidence' $(t_1/t)^2 + (t_2/t)^2 + \ldots + (t_n/t)^2$ might be a reasonable measure of how much one is concentrating one's efforts or spreading one's efforts. This could be a measure of the capacity to concentrate and therefore fitness for work. For the author this measure is now much less than before getting schizophrenia.

<u>Maintaining Insight with the Help of A Little Mathematics</u>

Abstract

I describe my experience of schizophrenia with special emphasis on some 'self-administered cognitive therapy', for delusions, based on Bayes' Theorem and subsequently Bayes' Rule. This technique has, I think, helped me maintain insight and could, I believe, also be used to combat various positive symptoms of psychosis in many other individuals, helping them gain or maintain insight.

Keywords: Delusions, Bayes' Theorem, Bayes' Rule.

Introduction

My experience of schizophrenia began in February 1999 when I had an acute psychotic episode which interrupted my mathematical research career. After losing my job, paranoid and in distress in a hotel far from home, I struck my head against a bath in an attempt to, as I believed at the time, wake myself up from a dream as I believed the unpleasant reality was not real. When some paramedics appeared suddenly this led to the delusion that I was now dead (as a result of hitting my head on the bath) and was being taken by them to hell (much as one character in the film Ghost (which I had seen years before) was).

Though I largely recovered from this episode, the delusion never went away entirely, becoming an 'over-valued idea'. Later in 1999 I had a relapse. The same delusion persisted and developed, with refinements of the delusional hypothesis of being dead into being dead and in hell or in a world that was changing gradually into hell. These delusions persisted for years, without me telling anyone about them, including a clinical psychologist I met with in 2000, as I believed that everyone might be a devil in disguise.

The delusions began to diminish in strength in 2001 (though I had retreated from the world to a large extent and was lying on my bed most of the day at this time and not taking my anti-psychotic medication). Taken to hospital in 2001, I was put on anti-psychotic medication again and an anti-depressant which helped lift my mood. This, along with a positive encounter with a friendly female patient in the clinic, helped to disprove my delusional hypotheses, and the delusions largely disappeared, to an extent greater than at any time since the first psychotic episode, but not completely. The casual mentioning of hell, death and related matters (which is ubiquitous in society though usually light-hearted) remained worrying to me, reminding me of my delusion and maintaining the delusion as an over-valued idea.

However, I intuitively began to dismiss the delusional hypotheses still further and in 2004 sought to strengthen this conviction as much as possible with the aid of mathematics, which I view as the most reliable arbiter of truth. Thinking about basic probability I realised that the mathematical result called Bayes' Theorem (see, e.g., [1, 2, 3]) could have something relevant to say about hypotheses, delusional or otherwise.

Bayes' Theorem and my use of it

Bayes' Theorem is a way of updating beliefs based on evidence that I was taught in my first year of an undergraduate maths degree. Let $P(A)$ denote the probability of A. Let $P(A|B)$ denote the probability of A given that B is true. Then Bayes' Theorem is as follows.

Theorem

Suppose we have some evidence E and are considering some hypotheses H_1, H_2, ... , H_n which are mutually exclusive and exhaustive. Then the probability of H_i given the evidence is given by

$P(H_i|E) = P(E|H_i)P(H_i) / [P(E|H_1)P(H_1) + \ldots + P(E|H_n)P(H_n)]$.

We may apply this to examine the probability of certain hypotheses I entertained. Let H_{hell} be the hypothesis that I am dead and in hell. Let H_{heaven} be the hypothesis that I am dead and in heaven. The only alternative hypothesis that I am prepared to consider is that I have paranoid schizophrenia or some other similar psychosis, which I denote by $H_{schizophrenia}$. I assume these three hypotheses are mutually exclusive, and they exhaust the possible hypotheses I am prepared to entertain. Also, let E be the experiences I have had since 1999.

Now I make subjective estimates for the probabilities concerned. First, I assign the prior probabilities (prior to the evidence) according to how I thought soon after the paramedics appeared. It is relatively easy to estimate P($H_{schizophrenia}$) since it is known that about 1 in 100 people gets schizophrenia, so I estimate this as 0.01. At the time, I knew almost nothing about madness, but I think I would have been willing to assign it this probability. However, I thought it very likely that I was dead when the paramedics came and probably going to hell, let's say twice as likely hell as heaven, so I assign P(H_{hell})=0.66 and P(H_{heaven})=0.33. This way the probabilities for the three hypotheses add up to one, as they should.

Now I consider what are called the likelihoods. Intuitively the probability of being in hell (or at least somewhere changing into hell) has seemed large at times, especially when bad events happen in the world (the saying 'going to hell in a handcart' comes to mind), but judging by how much has seemed normal in the period covered by E, I consider P(E|H_{hell}) to be very small, say 1 in a million. Whilst I have much to be thankful for, again I assign P(E|H_{heaven}) to be 1 in a million. P(E|$H_{schizophrenia}$) would have to be quite large (though I don't think I have auditory or visual hallucinations) so on balance I go for the middling figure of 0.5. Substituting these values into Bayes' Theorem, we obtain P(H_{hell}|E) ~ 1/7577, P(H_{heaven}|E) ~ 1/15154 and P($H_{schizophrenia}$|E) ~ 0.9998 to 4 decimal places. Thus, by my reckoning, the posterior probability that I have schizophrenia or some other similar psychosis is approximately 99.98%, despite my strongly believing other-worldly hypotheses in the prior.

However, one period's posterior is the next period's prior, and in each week since writing the above I have had further experiences, let us call some typical week's experiences E_2 say. During this time one might have minor problems, such as a cold, which is not my idea of heaven, so I reckon P(E_2|H_{heaven})=1/1000. Similarly, I expect things would be much worse if I was in hell, so I reckon P(E_2|H_{hell})=1/1000. I generally experience a pretty average time for a schizophrenic I suppose, so again I go for $P(E_2|H_{schizophrenia})=0.5$. Updating the old posterior probabilities using the new likelihoods and Bayes' Theorem we now have

$P(H_{hell}|E,E_2) \sim 1/3787744$, $P(H_{heaven}|E,E_2) \sim 1/7575488$ and $P(H_{schizophrenia}|E,E_2) \sim 0.9999996$ to 7 decimal places. So after including a single week's further evidence I am now even more certain that there is something 'wrong' with me, rather than with the world. (Note that this process of updating probabilities could be done using Bayes Theorem every so often, say after each week, further bolstering $H_{schizophrenia}$ and undermining H_{heaven} and H_{hell} and thus giving very good and fairly robust insight.)

This conclusion agrees with my official diagnosis, by the psychiatrists, of paranoid schizophrenia.

Bayes' Rule and my use of it

I had forgotten about Bayes' Rule till fairly recently, but it makes what is going on much clearer if you are mathematically minded and the calculations much simpler, so I will now describe the rule.

Given hypotheses H_1, H_2 and event E, let $O(H_1 : H_2)$ denote the prior odds of $H_1:H_2$. Then $O(H_1 : H_2)=P(H_1)/P(H_2)$. Let $O(H_1 : H_2|E)$ denote the posterior odds of $H_1:H_2$ given E. Then $O(H_1 : H_2|E)=P(H_1|E)/P(H_2|E)$. Let $L(H_1 : H_2|E)$ denote what is called the Bayes factor or likelihood ratio. Then $L(H_1 : H_2|E) = P(E|H_1)/P(E|H_2)$.

Bayes' rule (see, e.g., [4]) states that the posterior odds of $H_1 : H_2$ given E are equal to the prior odds of $H_1 : H_2$ multiplied by the Bayes factor, i.e.:

$O(H_1 : H_2|E) = L(H_1 : H_2|E) \, O(H_1 : H_2)$.

Suppose I entertain just two hypotheses, H_p denoting the hypothesis that I have psychosis and H_{np} denoting all other considered explanations (involving no psychosis - here including just the hypothesis of being dead and in hell or heaven). Then the odds prior to considering any evidence, $O(H_p : H_{np})$, could be 1/100 due to feeling fairly convinced of being dead and in heaven or hell. However, looking back over a moderately substantial period of time (such as the years from 1999 to 2004), with E denoting events in that period, the Bayes factor $P(E|H_p)/P(E|H_{np})$ is going to be very large, perhaps 1 million, say, as the probability of events given the psychosis is so enormously much higher than under the 'I have no psychosis' hypothesis (the figures could be 0.5 and 0.0000005 respectively, for example). Thus, the posterior odds in this case would be 1/100 times 1,000,000 = 10,000. Using the last posterior as the prior for further updating of the odds given further events, one now starts with prior odds of 10,000 and will multiply them by another large Bayes factor, say 1000, to get odds 10,000,000. The Bayes factor will always be greater than 1 providing one is reasonably sane when estimating it and recent experiences have not been too catastrophic, so it is easy to see that if one continues to live in a reasonably normal way the odds will increase and the delusional hypothesis can hopefully be dismissed for all practical purposes quite soon.

As one can see the calculation needed to update beliefs after each period of events is much simpler with Bayes' Rule than with Bayes' Theorem, so if one is willing to use Bayes' Rule things are easier. However, some of the detail is slightly hidden in the analysis above, in particular the decisions over what Bayes' factors to use, so to make everything explicit and really get to the bottom of things I now consider Bayes' Rule for a *series* of events or periods of experiences, one after the other.

This next section is quite 'technical', as some might say, and some readers may, without much loss, skip it.

Bayes' Rule for a series of events

We start with a series of three events and then generalise the analysis to arbitrarily many events.

Let the events be E_1 followed by E_2 followed by E_3. Let $E \cap F$ denote the event that both events E and F happen, and $E \cap F \cap G$ denote the event that events E, F and G all happen.

$O(H_1 : H_2 | E_1 \cap E_2 \cap E_3)$ is defined to be:

$$\frac{P(H_1 | E_1 \cap E_2 \cap E_3)}{P(H_2 | E_1 \cap E_2 \cap E_3)}$$

$$= \frac{P(H_1 \cap E_1 \cap E_2 \cap E_3)/P(E_1 \cap E_2 \cap E_3)}{P(H_2 \cap E_1 \cap E_2 \cap E_3)/(P(E_1 \cap E_2 \cap E_3)} \quad \text{(by definition of conditional probability)}$$

$$= \frac{P(H_1 \cap E_1 \cap E_2 \cap E_3)}{P(H_2 \cap E_1 \cap E_2 \cap E_3)} \quad \text{(simplifying)}$$

$$= \frac{P(E_3 | H_1 \cap E_1 \cap E_2)P(H_1 \cap E_1 \cap E_2)}{P(E_3 | H_2 \cap E_1 \cap E_2)P(H_2 \cap E_1 \cap E_2)} \quad \text{('peeling off' } E_3 \text{ by definition of conditional probability)}$$

$$= \frac{P(E_3 | H_1 \cap E_1 \cap E_2)P(E_2 | H_1 \cap E_1)P(H_1 \cap E_1)}{P(E_3 | H_2 \cap E_1 \cap E_2)P(E_2 | H_2 \cap E_1)P(H_2 \cap E_1)} \quad \text{(ditto with } E_2\text{)}$$

$$= \frac{P(E_3 | H_1 \cap E_1 \cap E_2)P(E_2 | H_1 \cap E_1)P(E_1 | H_1)P(H_1)}{P(E_3 | H_2 \cap E_1 \cap E_2)P(E_2 | H_2 \cap E_1)P(E_1 | H_2)P(H_2)} \quad \text{(ditto with } E_1\text{)}$$

$$= L(H_1:H_2,3)L(H_1:H_2,2)L(H_1:H_2,1)O(H_1:H_2),$$

where:

$$L(H_1:H_2,n) = \frac{P(E_n|H_1 \cap E_1 \cap E_2 \cap ... \cap E_{n-1})}{P(E_n|H_2 \cap E_1 \cap E_2 \cap ... \cap E_{n-1})}. \quad (*)$$

For a general number of events, n,

$O(H_1 : H_2|E_1 \cap E_2 \cap ... \cap E_{n-1} \cap E_n)$

$$= L(H_1:H_2,n)L(H_1:H_2,n-1)...L(H_1:H_2,2)L(H_1:H_2,1)O(H_1:H_2)$$

,

and

$$O(H_1:H_2|E_1 \cap ... \cap E_n) = L(H_1:H_2,n)O(H_1:H_2|E_1 \cap ... \cap E_{n-1}).$$
(**)

Now, examining equation (*) we see that the right-hand-side is just the ratio of the chances of observing the latest event given all the previous events under the two competing hypotheses. If $H_1 = H_p$ and $H_2 = H_{np}$ then the right-hand-side of (*) should exceed one so the left-hand-side of (**) will grow as n increases.

Of course, one could be being lulled into a false sense of security, prior to a nasty surprise, like in the 'Tea-breaks over, back on your heads' joke about hell (see [5]), but that will seem increasingly unlikely.

Thus from (**), $O(H_p : H_{np}|E_1 \cap E_2 \cap ... \cap E_{n-1} \cap E_n)$ will increase as time passes and n increases, and so confidence in the diagnosis of schizophrenia will increase.

Discussion

Cognitive therapy for delusions, voices and paranoia is already practised (see, e.g., [6]). However, I could not benefit much from any therapy as I did not tell anyone about the delusions I entertained until I had largely dismissed them - although I was seen by a clinical psychologist several times in 2000 I told him nothing about my thoughts as I thought he would dismiss them as false if I was dead and in hell as he would want to trick me. I suppose I had to dismiss the delusions myself before trusting some people with my thoughts. Perhaps following the nice encounter in the clinic in 2001 my brain subconsciously applied Bayesian analysis (see [7]). However, I think I want all the support I can get from mathematics to help me stay functioning reasonably well despite fairly frequent residual symptoms, and the mathematics explained here helps me be confident of my diagnosis and therefore maintain insight.

Hopefully if I stay on medication I won't have another relapse and I can continue to quickly dismiss the delusions I often briefly entertain after mishearing what's said or thinking it's directed at me (delusions of reference), with my strong conviction that it's the schizophrenia that's to blame.

I gradually reduced my anti-psychotic in three stages between 2007 and 2009 (from 400mg to 350mg, then 325mg and finally 300mg) and since 2014 I have been off my anti-depressant, without significant problems. In 2009, following the medication reductions, I gave an hour-and-a-half-long mathematical seminar. It was one of the greatest days of my life. Since 2010 I have finished and published four books on www.lulu.com under my pseudonym Chris O Hapinez (an anagram of guess what!), including an autobiography ('Everyone's A Devil In Disguise'), a work of non-fiction about mental illness ('A Handbook For Schizophrenics') and two collections of poetry and short prose ('The Woes Of A Schizophrenic' (sometimes downbeat) and 'Springtime For Schizophrenics' (very much upbeat)). I also published two collections of poetry and a book of paintings under my own name. Following a further medication reduction in 2018 to 287.5mg I have regularly conducted mathematical research for the first time since I acquired my illness, and read ten mathematical textbooks (previously I had been reading mostly the (relatively simple) popular science maths books) and published a light-hearted book of the mathematical popular science genre and another book of poetry. The latter medication reduction (though by only about 4%) has transformed my life for the better and re-awoken me mathematically. A further reduction in medication (of not much more than 1%) to 283.33mg in 2020 resulted in still more activity mathematically, conducting mathematical research more consistently and starting a collaboration with an academic mathematician, as well as publishing another book of poetry.

In a way, gaining insight into one's condition of psychosis (in my case schizophrenia) could be termed a 'P versus NP' problem of psychiatry (with the competing hypotheses H_p and H_{np}) somewhat like the famous (but very different) mathematics/computer science problem of 'P versus NP' - both being very important in their field.

I hope that a similar use of Bayes' Theorem or Bayes' Rule (though in general with different figures and hypotheses) could help many other mathematically-minded schizophrenics or people with psychosis reach a similar conclusion and gain insight or shore up existing insight into their condition, whether their symptoms are delusions, hearing voices, visual hallucinations or anything else.

References

[1] R. Swinburne, editor. *Bayes's Theorem*. Oxford University Press, Oxford, 2002.

[2] Bayesian Inference. https://en.wikipedia.org/wiki/Bayesian_inference.

[3] Bayes' theorem. https://en.wikipedia.org/wiki/Bayes'_theorem.

[4] Bayes' Rule. https://en.wikipedia.org/wiki/Bayes'_rule.

[5] Picking a punishment. www.ahajokes.com/hea14.html

[6] P. Chadwick, M. Birchwood, and P. Trower. *Cognitive Therapy for Delusions, Voices and Paranoia.* John Wiley and Sons, Chichester, 1996.

[7] R. Bain. *Are our brains Bayesian?* Significance, 13(4), 14-19, 2016.

The Law

See:

Mental Health Act 1983 Code of Practice: 2008 Revision by the Department of Health Stationery Office, ISBN 9780113228096, £16.50.

You may be able to get free, confidential legal advice and assistance from a local Law Centre. See http://www.lawcentres.org.uk/ for more information.

The Madness and Genius/Creativity Connection

"There is no great genius without a tincture of madness" – Seneca, 1st century AD.

"Great wits are sure to madness near allied, and thin partitions do their bounds divide" – John Dryden, 1681.

The writer Jack Kerouac and mathematician John Forbes Nash Jr suffered from schizophrenia. John Forbes Nash Jr won a Nobel Prize in Economics for his work in the mathematical field of Game Theory, and the Abel Prize (the equivalent of the Nobel Prize in Mathematics).

Many geniuses have had, or are suspected to have had, bipolar disorder, e.g., Beethoven.

From The Guardian, 9.6.15, page 1: "In a large study published yesterday, scientists in Iceland say genetic factors that raise the risk of bipolar disorder and schizophrenia are found more often in people in creative professions. Painters, musicians, writers and dancers were, on average, 25% more likely to carry the gene variants than those in professions the scientists judged to be less creative – among them farmers, manual labourers and salespeople."

Therapeutic Art

From Department for Health and Arts Council, 'A prospectus for arts and health', 2007:

"Arts can make a significant contribution to improving health and wellbeing of patients, service users and carers."

Treatment for Schizophrenia

From New Scientist, 8.2.14, pages 32-35:

"Although people need to be taken off their drugs slowly and carefully to avoid a relapse, it looks as though outcomes are better in the long run if medication is kept to a minimum."

"They (antipsychotics) can also make people feel both unhappy and highly agitated, a potentially lethal combination, says psychiatrist David Healy, head of the North Wales Department of Psychological Medicine, Bangor, UK. His study of historical records from a Welsh mental hospital showed that 100 years ago people with schizophrenia were no more likely to kill themselves than the general population. This suggests it is modern drugs that cause schizophrenia's high suicide rate, he says."

"More importantly, those in the stopping medication group (minimal or no drugs) had more than double the chance of achieving what psychiatrists call "functional recovery" – 40 versus 18 percent (JAMA Psychiatry, vol 70, p. 913). In other words, even though they might have occasional symptoms, they could hold down jobs and look after themselves."

"Along with others, Moncrieff believes antipsychotics may simply be another version of the tranquillisers used back in the 1950s."

"It is possible for people to have ongoing symptoms and yet hold down a job," says Max Birchwood.

Treatment without Drugs

Rufus May, a clinical psychologist in the NHS who had been diagnosed as schizophrenic himself, treats patients without drugs, which he says make you stupid.

Such treatments include Counselling, Psychotherapy and talking with a Clinical Psychologist – see also the topics Cognitive Remediation Therapy and Cognitive Behavioural Therapy in this book.

See www.rufusmay.com .

From The Daily Mirror, 11.12.15:

"A more holistic approach is favoured in Australia and Scandinavia and now a rigorous US study has defined a programme where the main remedy is just talking. Yes, talk therapy. When it works, it allows much lower doses of those mind-numbing antipsychotic drugs."

Transcranial Magnetic Stimulation (TMS) may be an effective treatment for some with schizophrenia – see Monash University Magazine, September 2016.

Open Dialogue

Originating in Finland in the 1980s, this relatively new approach has been trialled in the UK recently, starting in 2017. See, e.g., https://www.kmpt.nhs.uk/information-and-advice/open-dialogue/ .

Understanding Schizophrenia

From The Observer, 12.11.17, Mental Health? It's in the mind and the body, too: "This month, British Scientists began testing a radical new approach to treating schizophrenia based on emerging evidence that it could be a disease of the immune system."

Universal Credit

Universal Credit has a number of flaws, not least the immoral 'Minimum Income Floor', which means that if you earn less from your own business in a month than the minimum income floor, then your money is not topped up and you may have to either starve/go into debt etc. or give up working!

University Life

The University of Bedfordshire has a Mental Health Advisor.

Nottingham Trent University has a mental-health adviser.

City University has a mental health and wellbeing support service and a mental health and wellbeing co-ordinator.

Websites on schizophrenia and other mental illnesses and quotes from the web

An interesting quote from the web which lays down the gauntlet to all schizophrenics is the following from http://www.maximumcrowe.net/maxcrowe_bminprint3.html (no longer accessible) which is *The Lost Years of a Nobel Laureate* By Sylvia Nasar, The New York Times, 1994:

Schizophrenia is often confused with manic depressive illness, the disease that afflicted Vincent Van Gogh, Virginia Woolf and a host of other geniuses. But that illness, primarily a disorder of mood rather than of thinking, typically arrives later in life. Sufferers can often hold high-level jobs and do extremely creative work between bouts. Schizophrenia, on the other hand, is too debilitating to co-exist with great accomplishment. Nijinsky, the Russian dancer, is one of the few known victims of schizophrenia other than Mr. Nash to have made his mark as a genius before the disease struck.

From http://pn.psychiatryonline.org/content/39/11/36.full (no longer accessible) 'In Families With Psychosis, The Numbers Tell a Story':

So it looks as though there may be a relationship between math talent and a risk of psychosis, Karlsson concluded.

General Mental Health Sites:

National Alliance on Mental Illness www.nami.org/Home

Mental Health America   www.mhanational.org

http://www.theguardian.com/society/mental-health

Very Well Mind www.verywellmind.com

American Psychiatric Association http://www.psychiatry.org/

http://www.mind.org.uk/

http://www.mentalhelp.net/

http://psychcentral.com/

Internet Mental Health (includes information on lots of medications)

http://www.mentalhealth.com/

http://www1.mhsanctuary.com/

http://www.kcl.ac.uk/ioppn

http://www.dorothyrowe.com.au/

www.criticalpsychiatry.co.uk

Schizoaffective Disorder:

http://www.schizoaffective.org/

http://www.schizoaffective.net/

Schizophrenia:

http://www.schizophrenia.com/

Ian Chovil's Homepage http://www.chovil.com/

Part of this very good site contained the following:

One of my visitors recommended *The Messenger* which is about Joan of Arc. I haven't seen it yet but I think she would probably have had bipolar disorder simply because she has become famous. There are probably quite a few saints who either had a form of epilepsy or bipolar disorder that didn't disable them as much as schizophrenia would have. John Nash is famous and he definitely had schizophrenia but he accomplished his Nobel Prize award winning work before he experienced his first psychosis. For the next thirty years or so he wasn't able to do very much at all. That is what often distinguishes schizophrenia from bipolar, the sheer disability associated with schizophrenia.

Perceptions Forum/Voices Forum http://www.voicesforum.org

Open the doors http://www.openthedoors.com/

http://www.schizophrenia-help.com/

http://psychcentral.com/schizophrenia

http://the-wife-of-a-schizophrenic.blogspot.com/

Manic Depression:

http://www.manicmoment.org/

http://www.bipolarbrain.com/

http://www.mdf.org.uk/

Bipolar Disorder News, Information and Support
http://www.pendulum.org/

Depression:

http://www.allaboutdepression.com/

http://www.depression.org.uk/

http://www.clinical-depression.co.uk/

http://www.depressionalliance.org/

http://www.depression-helper.com/

http://www.ifred.org/

http://www.mcmanweb.com/

http://www.samaritans.org/

http://www.suicidal.com/

Depression and Bipolar Support Alliance
www.dbsalliance.org

Weight gain with antipsychotics

Source unknown.

Here is a table that may be of interest:

Risk of weight gain	Drug
Very high	Clozapine
High	Olanzapine
	Thioridazine
	Zotepine
Medium	Chlorpromazine
	Risperidone
	Thioxanthines
	Quetiapine
Low	Amisulpride/sulpiride
	Butyrophenones
	Pimozide
	Piperazine phenothiazines
Very low	Ziprasidone

Work Capability Assessments

Work Capability Assessments (WCA) as devised by the Department for Work and Pensions (DWP) have been criticised by GPs and at least one Court. See, e.g., *GPS call for work capability assessment to be scrapped*, The Guardian, 23.5.12 and *Fitness-for-work tests unfair on people with mental health problems, court says*, The Guardian, 22.5.13.

What can aid or prevent recovery

From Whole Life, Whole Systems, Luton & Bedford – March 2004, Feedback from user involvement groups:

What can aid recovery?

Relationships/Social

Support from family and friends

Love and friendships

Conversations and being listened to

Drop-In centres/social groups

Good day care

Support with social integration

Trips out/generally something to look forward to

Occupation

Work – in particular part-time work

Hobbies and keeping busy

Exercise

Giving something back to the community

Being usefully occupied – meaningful voluntary or paid work

Supported employment

College courses

Practical Issues

Correct benefits

Better benefit advice

Local assessment (specific complaint from Bedford group who have to travel to Luton for benefits assessment)

Practical support for specific issues, i.e., learning to clean, cook, look after yourself etc.

Good accommodation

Wider range of accommodation

More group homes and supported accommodation

Advice

Better public transport

Services outside of Bedford

Comprehensive information about what is available

Treatments/Therapy

Workshop therapies

Relaxation/music

Access to therapeutic groups

Reducing drug and alcohol dependency

Balanced diet

Good sleeping pattern

Emotional support – out of hours if needed

Access to psychotherapy

Education about mental health issues

Reliable statutory support

Respect – particularly from psychiatrists

Psychiatrists having more time for consultations

More to do when in hospital

Working together with statutory staff

Support from GPs

More privacy – not being expected to tell support workers everything

Right level of medication/being relatively free of symptoms

Combination and range of services and treatment – home, respite, hospital

More respite care

Care planning related to the recovery model

Friendships on a professional basis

Staff respecting users as individuals

Better NHS complaints procedure

General Wellbeing

Self-confidence

Time and space

Learning to live with an illness

Taking control over your life/independence

To feel comfortable and satisfied with yourself

Having a voice and opinion

Stability

Regular routine

Losing a label

Leading a "normal" life

Integration

Peace of mind and enjoying life

Living healthily

Wider Social Issues

Racial Harmony

Education on mental health issues

Reduction of stigma in society

Feeling safe – less violence in towns and cities

Less crime and less prosecution

Sympathetic employers

<u>What can prevent recovery?</u>

Relationships/Social

Isolation/loneliness/boredom

Losing contact with family and friends

Poor understanding of family and friends

No "normal" friendships

Occupation

Unemployment

Poor Government employment schemes

Only menial work available

No progression in employment

Benefits system in relation to employment

Practical Issues

Lack of money/the benefits system

Poor accommodation

Treatments/Therapies

Misdiagnosis

Being labelled or wrongly labelled

Lack of choice and freedom

Arrogance/ignorance of staff

Poor quality staff

Lack of mutual trust

Poor respite care

Lack of comprehensive services

Poor assessment procedures

Incorrect medication

Failure to take medication

Poor continuity of psychiatric and day care support

Too many staff changes

No real qualitative measures of care

No standardised method of referral (particularly from primary care sources)

Poor GP support

Poor understanding of illness/medication and its effects

Poor symptom control

Inadequate support in hospital and when leaving hospital

Too much medication and not enough therapies in hospital

GPs missing physical problems

General Wellbeing

Apathy

Lack of self-respect and self-esteem

Lack of confidence

Lack of faith

Poor diet

Denial of problem

Alcohol and drugs

Lack of understanding of illness and recovery

Grief

Peer pressure

Wider Social Issues

Media portrayal

Prejudice

Public ignorance and preconceptions

What some psychology students were taught about schizophrenia

From SAGB Newsletter, Spring 2007:

"Schizophrenia, we were taught, was probably the worst of all mental illnesses." – Roz Hewitt, the author of *Moving On: A guide to good health and recovery for people with a diagnosis of schizophrenia.*

Printed in Great Britain
by Amazon